Stop Sciatica Now

Third Edition

Help Yourself
Eliminate Back and Leg Pain

by Pamela Kihm

PainFreeChoices®
P.O. Box 7078, Evanston, IL 60204–7078
www.painfreechoices.com

First Edition Copyright © 2003 by Pamela Kihm
Revised Edition Copyright © 2006 by Pamela Kihm
Third Edition Copyright © 2009 by Pamela Kihm

All rights reserved. No part of this book can be reproduced by any means for any purpose without the express written permission of Pamela Kihm.

ISBN 0-9779102-0-2

7th printing redesign: Matthew Doherty, Matthew Doherty Design, Evanston, Il.
Third Edition print edit: Donnelly J. Barclay, May Ruth Spitzer
Revised Edition format edit: John Urish
First Printing format: Marcia Coulter
Illustrator: Flora Hill
Medical illustrations: John Bauer, H.V. Carter
Photography: Rachel Kuly

Feldenkrais®, *Feldenkrais Method®*, *Awareness Through Movement®*, and *Functional Integration®* are registered service marks of the *Feldenkrais Guild®* of North America.

Guild Certified Feldenkrais Teacher^{CM} and *Guild Certified Feldenkrais Practitioner^{CM}* are certification marks of the *Feldenkrais Guild®* of North America.

Many of the designations used by manufacturers and sellers to distinguish their products are claimed as trademarks. Where those designations appear in this book and PainFreeChoices® was aware of the trademark claim, the designation is followed by the following symbol: ®.

The information contained in this book is not intended to replace regular medical checkups. No book can possibly replace the services of a health care provider who knows you personally.

Publisher
PainFreeChoices®
P. O. Box 7078 Evanston, IL 60204-7078
www.painfreechoices.com

Table of Contents

1	Introduction	1
2	Your Sciatic Nerve Network	7
3	Reorganize Skeletally	13
4	Gentle Exercises To Reduce Pain	23
5	Constructive Fidgeting	35
6	More Self-Help Techniques	43
7	Moving Through Your Day	53
8	Walking Can Be Therapeutic	67
9	Travel Comfortably	75
10	Resume Activities Confidently	83
	About the Author	93
	Glossary	94
	Index of Lessons	96

Additional books by Pamela Kihm

Walking: Nature's Perfect Exercise

Relax Your Back With a Roller

www.painfreechoices.com

for more books

Foreword

Whatever the cause of your sciatica, chances are very good that you can reduce your own pain by following the advice in this book based on the *Feldenkrais Method*® of Somatic Education.

> The human body is a marvelously complex machine, and its musculo-skeletal system permits a remarkable range of movement. However, we are seldom fully aware of exactly what we do and how we do it. Often we unknowingly injure ourselves, but fortunately our bodies have a wonderful potential for self-healing. Participation in weekly *Feldenkrais Method*® *Awareness Through Movement*® classes has helped me to learn to re-educate myself, so that I can move more comfortably without pain and without undue limitations. Recently when I developed unexplained sciatic pain, several individual Feldenkrais sessions and continuing classes with Pamela Kihm enabled me to resolve the problem in a relatively short time. Mobility is essential to health, and *Feldenkrais* can be of great help to older people in maintaining their mobility. *Feldenkrais* principles should be included in the curriculum of every medical school.
>
> William B. Spriegel, M.D

1 Introduction

You—and you alone—make the moment-to-moment everyday decisions about how you sit, stand, and move. To prevent recurring bouts of sciatica and the need for pain medications, you must become the most active partner of your health care team.

How This Book Can Help You

Stop Sciatica Now explains how:

➢ Minor changes in your usual ways of sitting, standing, and walking can stop irritating your sciatic nerves and start the healing process.

➢ Habitually tensing your muscles excessively affects your sciatic nerves profoundly.

➢ When you position your skeleton effectively, your muscles don't have to tighten excessively.

Stop Sciatica Now shows you how to:

➢ Use what you already have in your everyday environment to relieve pain and prevent sciatica flare-ups.

➢ Become more aware of how you are positioning your body.

➢ Ward off future sciatica flare-ups through healthful movement choices and through gentle preventive maintenance exercises.

This book, which is based on the *Feldenkrais Method* of Somatic Education, will widen your options for moving in healthful ways.

There are scores of examples where the *Feldenkrais Method* of Somatic Education has greatly improved people's quality of movement. To quote Dr. John Chester, a retired orthopedic surgeon who has been part of some *Feldenkrais* trainings:

> *Many members of the medical community have seen the value of the* Feldenkrais Method *in improving their patients' lives and sometimes the underlying medical condition.*

Isadora, a client of mine who continued her social work practice into her eighties:

> *I was running to the chiropractor, osteopath, and physiotherapist. They were correcting the misalignments, but not teaching me how to avoid them. Now, with this new knowledge, I usually can work them out by myself. Most of all I have become pain free, and have a sense of control over my body.*

All the anatomical, medical, and special-use terms in this book are defined in the Glossary.

About This Chapter

This chapter includes the following:

➢ A brief history of Dr. Moshe Feldenkrais, physicist and developer of the *Feldenkrais Method*® of Somatic Education.

➢ An easy-to-do exercise so you can demonstrate for yourself how moving with skeletal awareness can increase your comfort and your effectiveness.

Introduction

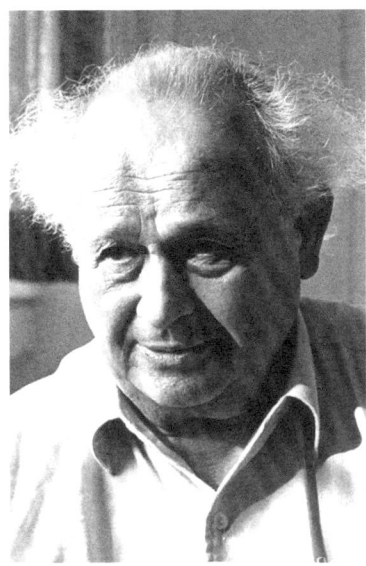

Courtesy of Feldenkrais Institute Tel Aviv, Israel

Feldenkrais – The Man and the Method

The information and exercises in this book are based on the *Feldenkrais Method®* of Somatic Education developed by Moshe Feldenkrais, DSc. Dr. Feldenkrais (1904-1984) had degrees in engineering as well as physics. The *Feldenkrais Method®* utilizes principles of physics, engineering, and biomechanics.

While playing soccer as a young man, Moshe Feldenkrais severely tore ligaments in his knee. Over the years, his pain and limp worsened and in the early 1940's, his long-term knee problem became intolerable. Doctors told him that there was only a 50% chance surgery could remove the pain and admitted that the surgery might lessen his ability to walk.

Moshe Feldenkrais chose not to have surgery. Instead, he applied his knowledge of engineering and biomechanics to his own body. Eventually he taught himself to walk without pain–and without a limp! He was able to participate fully in his very active life.

How Dr. Feldenkrais Eliminated His Own Pain

- He stopped forcing himself through the pain and, instead, paid attention to how he was moving when his pain was not as severe.

- He discovered that his skeletal positioning made the difference between movement that caused pain and movement that caused no pain.

Others saw what Moshe Feldenkrais had accomplished for himself and that he could help other people move more comfortably in spite of a wide variety of problems. They began to ask him to help their friends and relatives. Moshe returned to Israel where he began to apply his unique skills full-time, and so the *Feldenkrais Method®* came into being.

In addition to his hands-on work with individuals (*Functional Integration®*), Dr. Feldenkrais developed group classes where he could talk people through movement (*Awareness Through Movement®*). Frequently three generations of a family would attend classes where 80 to over 100 people participated.

Eventually Moshe Feldenkrais trained others to carry on his work of helping clients move more comfortably and effectively. The first professional training for *Feldenkrais® Practitioners* in the United States was completed in 1977, so this method is relatively new to this country. To date, there are about 3,000 *Feldenkrais Practitioners* worldwide.

Increasing Options

Feldenkrais Practitioners help clients discover many options beyond their existing habits of movement. The client can then choose to move in ways that eliminate pain and also improve coordination, flexibility, and balance.

Much is accomplished during a *Feldenkrais* session, but it's not the practitioner "fixing" the client and then telling the client to "hold" the adjustment. Clients participate and take what they learn into the rest of their lives.

We can use the analogy of a weight-loss program. If you pay to have healthful meals with the correct number of calories provided for a set period of time, you will shed pounds; however, unless you change life patterns of eating and exercise, the pounds will probably return.

As you read this book, you will learn how to take better care of yourself by moving in ways that are in your own best interest.

Feldenkrais Professional Training

To become certified as a *Feldenkrais Practitioner*, candidates must attend over 800 hours of classroom training and pass a certification test. In addition, they must annually complete twenty hours of continuing education in order to be re-certified every two years.

During the *Feldenkrais Professional Training*, *Feldenkrais Practitioners* become very aware of the muscular and nervous systems as well as the skeletal system. However, this book focuses on the skeleton because **the way a person is positioning and moving his or her skeleton is key to eliminating sciatic nerve pain.**

Touch Your Toes With More Comfort and Ease

This awareness exercise is designed to help you experience how the position of your skeleton can either hinder or improve the effectiveness and comfort of your movement.

Experiment to discover if the position of your skeleton can determine how hard—or how easy—it is to tie your shoes.

Equipment needed: a chair or bench

1. Sit on a chair or bench with your feet flat on the floor, a comfortable distance apart.

    Make sure that your knees are as far apart as your feet.

2. If necessary, loosen the clothing around your waist.

3. Reach toward your foot with one hand and then come back up to your original position.

    Did you round your back, caving in your chest? Or, did you bend forward from your hip joints?

To discover whether you rounded your back or bent forward through your hip joints, continue with the following steps.

4. Put the fingertips of one hand in the fold where your leg connects to the rest of your body. Then, with your fingertips still in the fold, bend forward and reach for your foot with the other hand.

    If you round your back, some space remains there when you reach for your toes.

    However, if you bend over by folding through your hip joints, that space closes up.

5. Reach for your foot by intentionally rounding your back. (This is what many people do every time they bend over to touch their toes.)

    What is the distance from your fingertips to your toes?

    Do you feel discomfort in your lower back?

6   Now reach for your foot again. But this time, fold forward where your legs are ball-and-socketed to your pelvis and let your back lengthen instead of round.

> Now what is the distance from your fingertips to your toes?

7   Alternate between Step 5 and Step 6.

> Which way allows your fingertips to get closer to your toes?
>
> Which way is more comfortable for your lower back and neck?

Explanation:

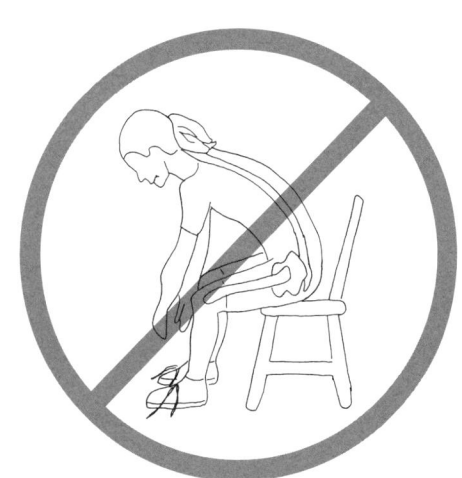

When you round your spine to touch your toes:

> The lower half of your spine actually goes backward.
>
> The bending forward happens in the upper back.
>
> Rounding your upper spine to touch your toes is not only inefficient; it can cause pain in your lower back.

When, instead of rounding your back you fold forward through your hip joints as you bend to touch your toes:

> The top of your hipbones and the top of your sacrum (the center back of your pelvis) tilt forward.
>
> Your whole spine tilts forward instead of just the top half of your spine curving like a hook.

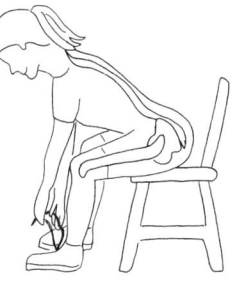

As you experiment with the awareness exercises in *Stop Sciatica Now*, you will discover that skeletal awareness can make you more comfortable and your movements more efficient. You will also discover that it takes no more effort to move with skeletal awareness than it does to mindlessly drag your bones and their connecting joints.

The fact is, in the split-second before you make any move, there is a moment where you subconsciously decide **how** you are going to move. This book will help you bring that split-second decision to the conscious level, so that you can move more effectively and won't damage your joints and the nerves that thread through those joints.

2 Your Sciatic Nerve Network

This chapter explains:

➢ How the sciatic nerve network threads through your skeleton, and

➢ How your body positioning affects your sciatic nerves.

The Skeletal Connection

The sciatic nerve network is a combination of two nerves, the tibial nerve and the common peroneal nerve. Both travel from your lower back down through your right leg and your left leg.

The tibial nerves connect to the right and the left of your spinal cord in five places through the following vertebrae: 4th and 5th lumbar and 1st, 2nd, and 3rd sacral.

The common peroneal nerves connect to the right and the left of your spinal cord in four places through the following vertebrae: the 4th and 5th lumbar and the 1st and 2nd sacral.

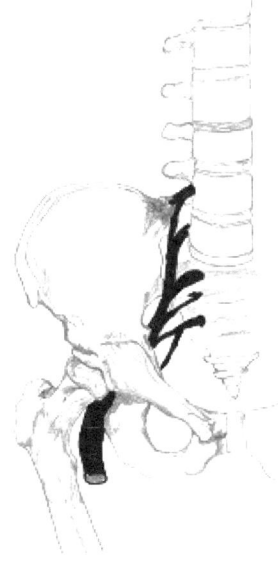

What this means to you: The way you position your lumbar vertebrae (lower back) and your sacrum (center back of your pelvis) affects your sciatic nerves. For example, slouching can irritate your sciatic nerves.

The drawing at left shows the sciatic nerve network threading through the lower back and femoral (hip) joint.

The tibial nerves thread from your spine through the bottom of each femoral joint (hip joint) where the "ball" of your femur (thigh bone) moves in the "socket" (acetabulum of your pelvis).

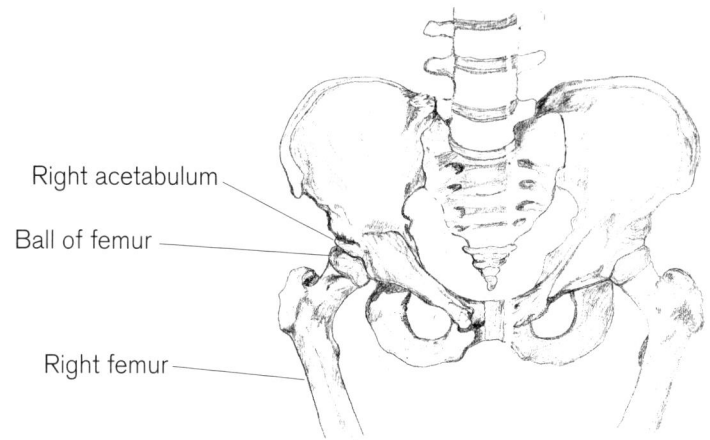

And, the common peroneal nerves pass in front of each sacroiliac joint where each ilium (hipbone) attaches to your sacrum (center back of your pelvis) and then threads under each femoral joint.

What this means to you: How you position and move your pelvis affects the comfort of your sciatic nerve network.

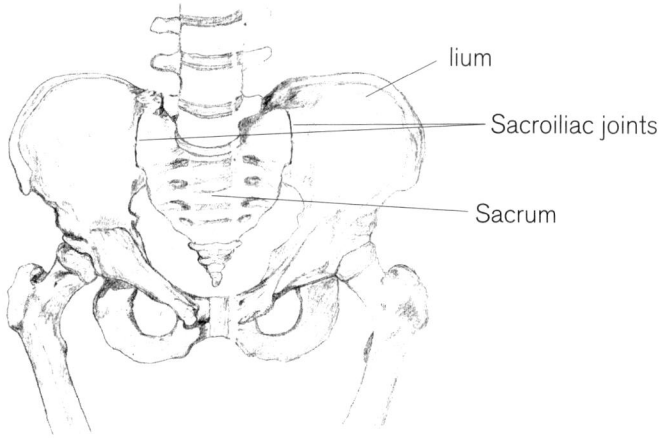

Your Sciatic Nerve Network

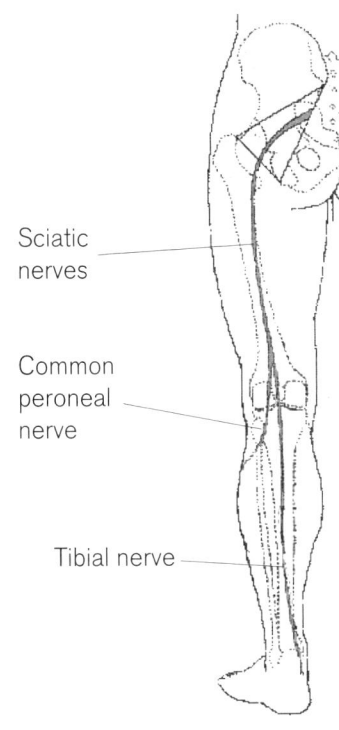

Sciatic nerves

Common peroneal nerve

Tibial nerve

The tibial nerves thread: down the center back of each thigh, behind each knee, down the back of each lower leg to the inner side of your ankle and heel, and through the arch to the underside of each foot.

What this means to you: If the edge of a chair or car seat puts pressure on the back of your thighs or knees it can irritate your sciatic nerves.

And, if you habitually hyper-extend your knees, you can irritate your sciatic nerves.

Note: Hyper-extended knees are so "straight" they actually bend a bit backward.

The common peroneal nerves:

➢ Branch away from the tibial nerve above each knee.

➢ Swerve down the outside of each knee and into the front of each lower leg just outside your tibia ("shin bone").

➢ Continue down through the outside of your ankle and into the top of your foot.

What this means to you: Habitually standing, walking, or sitting with your feet rolled outward or inward can irritate your sciatic nerves.

Note: To find out if you habitually roll your feet, check the wear pattern on the heels of your shoes

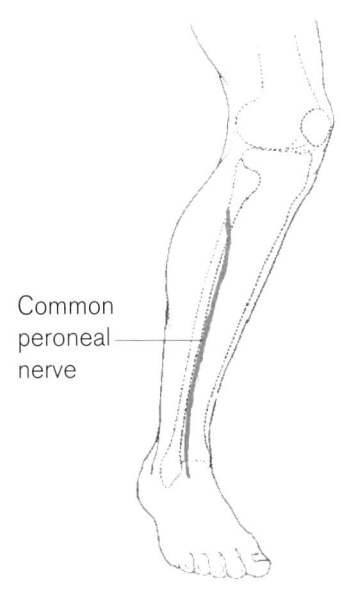

Common peroneal nerve

Both the tibial and common peroneal nerves weave between and under the powerful gluteus and piriformis muscles in your buttocks and thighs.

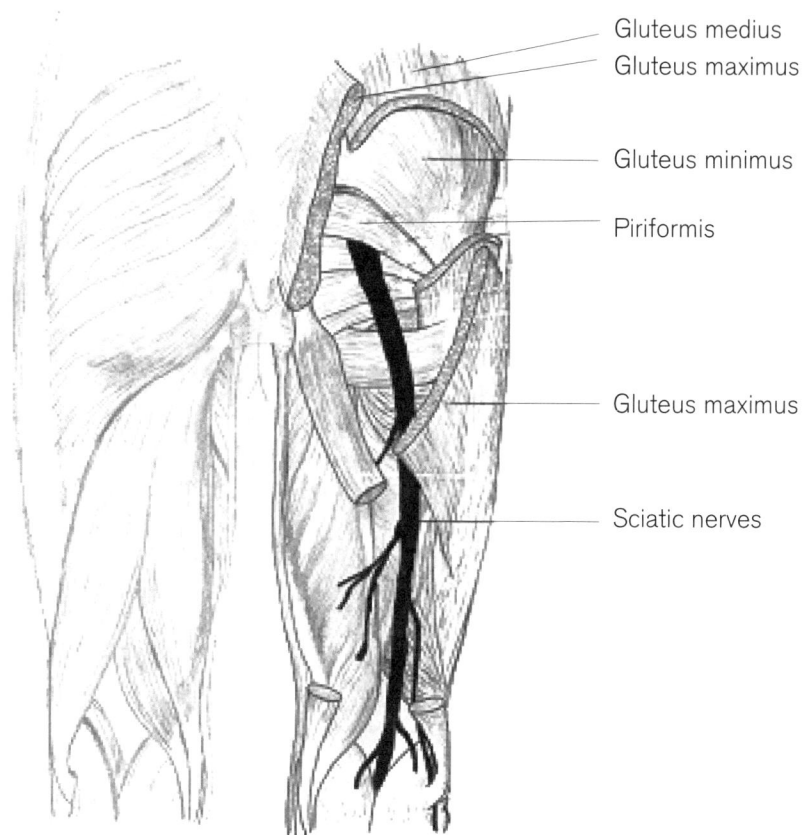

What this means to you: Habitually tightening the muscles through the buttocks and thighs can irritate your sciatic nerve network.

Habitually flattening away the natural lumbar curve of your lower back can irritate your sciatic nerve.

Habitually tightening your muscles so that your coccyx (tailbone) sinks under you can irritate your sciatic nerve.

Important: When you continually contract your muscles, whether to "flatten your stomach" or to guard against pain, the contracted muscles crowd the vessels that transport oxygen-rich blood. Oxygen deprivation can actually cause pain. Injured or irritated parts of your body need more oxygen to heal, not less.

Compounding The Problem

Many in the medical community still instruct patients with lower back and sciatic nerve pain to flatten their backs when standing. Many patients compound the problem by interpreting the instruction to "strengthen abdominal muscles" to mean "tighten abdominal muscles *all day long*."

Unfortunately health columns in newspapers and magazines still occasionally print instructions to flatten the whole back against the wall for ideal posture. Sometime when you're feeling good enough for a **brief** experiment, flatten your back against the wall and then try to walk with your back in that position. (It may feel familiar, but familiar isn't necessarily healthful.)

Walking with your back flattened will aggravate sciatica, not eliminate it.

Flattening your lower back tilts your femoral joints forward and your sacroiliac joints backward. It also squishes the discs (cushions) between each lumbar vertebra.

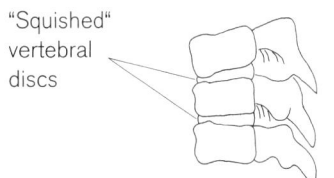

"Squished" vertebral discs

Feldenkrais Anticipated Ergonomic Principles

Today ergonomics experts recognize the importance of the human lumbar curve. They are perfecting ways to encourage you to have a lumbar curve while driving your car and working at your computer.

Dr. Feldenkrais recognized that human beings were meant to have a lumbar curve **when standing as well as when sitting**. When you flatten away your lumbar curve —whether consciously or subconsciously—your muscles work overtime, possibly irritating your sciatic nerve network.

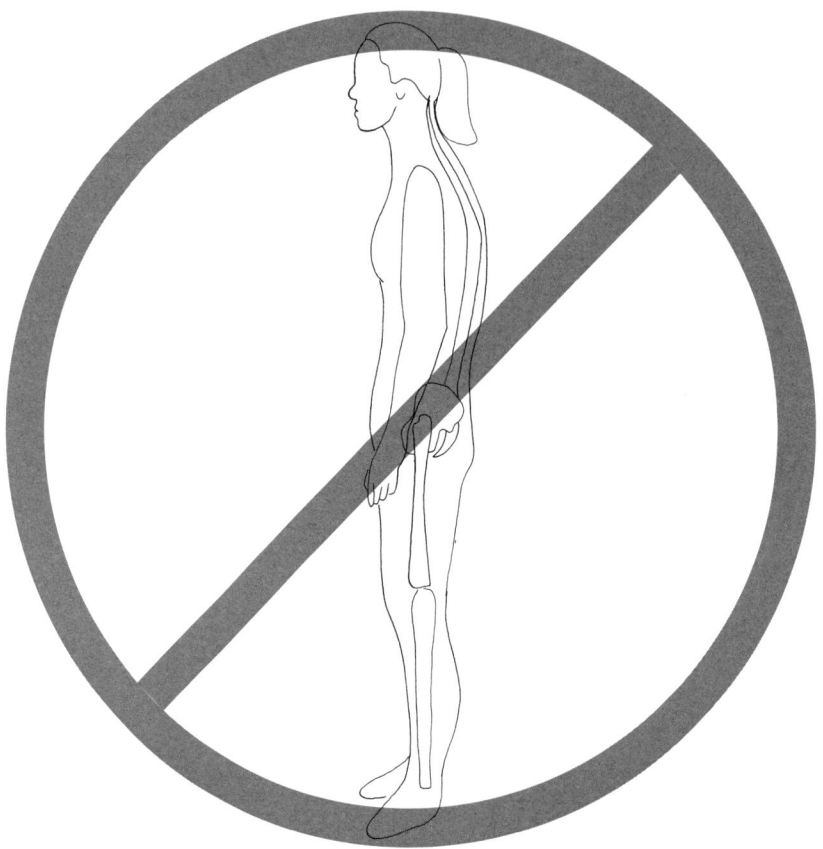

Summary

➢ Flattening away the natural lumbar curve of your lower back can irritate your sciatic nerves.

➢ Tightening your glutei muscles so that your coccyx sinks under you can irritate your sciatic nerves.

➢ Contracting, instead of lengthening, your abdominal muscles while you stand or walk can irritate your sciatic nerves.

➢ Hyper-extending your knees (knees actually move backward from neutral) can irritate your sciatic nerves.

3 Reorganize Skeletally

Sciatica is not a disease but a collection of symptoms frequently resulting from a less than ideal use of your body. Your pain is telling you to do something differently so you don't keep hurting yourself.

Don't ignore your pain. You know how pain shouts at you to pull your hand away from that hot stove. If you listen, even a small amount of discomfort tells you, "Position your body differently! Move in a different way!"

Gain and Maintain Posture From The Bottom Up

There's an easier, more comfortable way to gain and maintain your posture than tightening your upper body and lower back. Think of your body as skeletally engineered. What's below is meant to support what's above. This is the opposite of maintaining your posture from the top down.

Example of posture from the top down

1. Sit in a chair with a firm seat.
2. Slouch the way you would at the computer or watching TV.
3. Use your muscles to pull your shoulders back (the way many people try to effect better posture).

> Is your head still forward, even though you pulled your shoulders back?

> Does this make your neck uncomfortable? (If you stay this way, you invite neck and shoulder problems as well as lower back problems.)

> Can you use your arms freely and efficiently when you pull your shoulders back to stay upright?

4   With your shoulders still pulled back, use your muscles to pull your head back over your body so that you *look* like you are "in good posture."

　　How comfortable is this?

　　Could you maintain this position for long without hurting?

　　Is your lower back *still* in a slouch even though you've pulled your upper body upward and backward?

　　Can you feel how hard your lower back muscles are working to help your upper body?

Example of gaining and maintaining posture from the bottom up

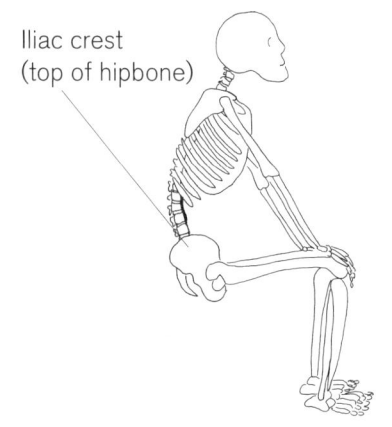
Iliac crest (top of hipbone)

1   Return to your starting position. That is, sit on a chair with a firm seat and slouch the way you did at the beginning of the experiment.

2   Put your hands on your iliac crests (the tops of your hipbones). Notice that when you slouch, the iliac crests tilt behind you.

　　The more you slouch, the further back your iliac crests tilt.

3   Rotate the top of your pelvis forward until your iliac crests point toward the ceiling instead of behind you.

　　➤ Did this take you into upright posture with less effort?

　　➤ Did you notice that your body moved into this upright posture without your shoulder muscles having to tense?

　　➤ Did your pelvis bring your head up over your body without your having to tense your neck muscles?

　　Are you now taller than a moment ago?

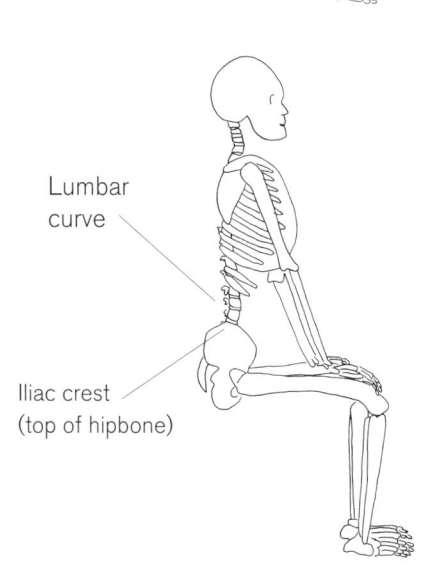
Lumbar curve
Iliac crest (top of hipbone)

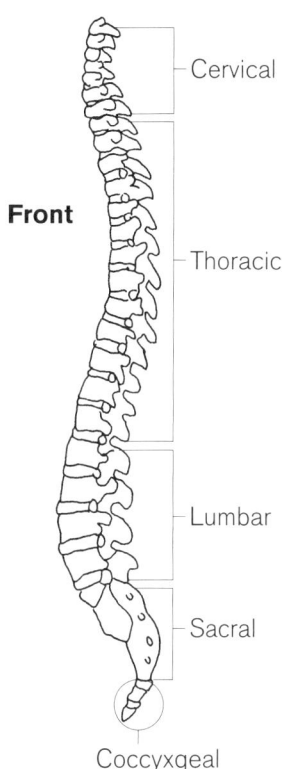

It's important to remember that your spine is a continuum, from the tip end of your coccyx (tailbone), through the sacrum (center back of your pelvis), to the top of your neck. Your pelvis is a powerful "handle" that you can use to effortlessly rearrange your whole spine to make your back, neck, and shoulders more comfortable.

Notice the spinal curves, including the lumbar curve, in a healthfully positioned spine. **We are meant to have those spinal curves.** Continually canceling out your lumbar curve can set you up for disc problems as well as sciatica.

Finding *Your* Most Healthful Posture

Moshe Feldenkrais had a profoundly simple way to help people find their most healthful posture when standing. He said, "*Pretend* you're about to jump up in the air." You don't have to *actually* jump—just move into position *as if to* jump. The changes in body-position that you have to make in order to jump are the exact changes needed for more comfortable and efficient standing and walking!

➤ If you're slouching, could you jump very high?

➤ If you kept your back positioned as if it were flattened against a wall, could you jump upward?

➤ If you kept your coccyx tucked under, could you jump upward?

➤ If you didn't allow some flexibility in your hip joints or your knees, could you jump?

➤ If your feet were wide apart and your knees were hyper-extended (too straight) could you jump upward?

All of the above prevents one from jumping upward; any of the above, if habitual, could irritate your sciatic nerve network.

The "jump" technique is very individual. Wherever you need to fold in order to jump is exactly where you need to let go of muscular rigidity to stop irritating your sciatic nerves.

In order to spring upward, a person has to "accordion pleat." You cannot accordion pleat through your femoral joints (where your leg meets your pelvis) if your coccyx is tucked under.

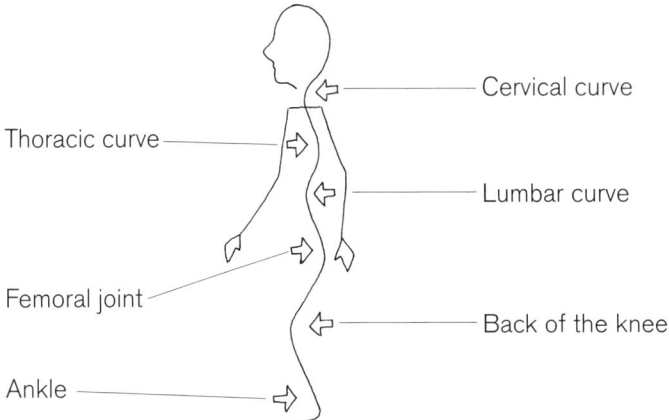

"Accordion pleating" is a technique to remind you where you need to eliminate rigidity in order to have good posture *and* be comfortable. You don't have to stand and walk with your knees dramatically bent; however, to keep sciatica at bay you do need to allow flexible bend-ability in your hip joints and knees.

When you first stand up, momentarily "accordion pleat" a little bit as if to jump, then softly lift up out of that without going all the way into old habits of coccyx tucking, back flattening, or knees hyper-extending.

Any time you feel discomfort while standing, momentarily "accordion pleat." Then, softly lift up through both your sternum and your sacrum so both the front and the back of your spine lengthen ***without losing your natural cervical, thoracic, and lumbar curves and the springiness in your hip, knee, and ankle joints.***

"Acture"

Dr. Feldenkrais didn't like to use the word posture. To him "posture" sounded statue-like—only useful when posing for a portrait. Instead, Dr. Feldenkrais coined the word "acture." In acture, the person is prepared for action. Moshe said that one is standing in acture when he or she doesn't have to make any adjustment before walking forward, backward, or to the side. The standing position that results from briefly accordion pleating or thinking "jump" is a perfect example of acture.

Sitting with one leg crossed over the other is *not* acture

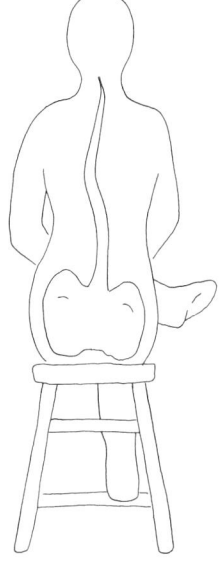

You have to uncross your legs before standing.

Your pelvis tilts when one leg crosses the other. (If flexibility in your hip joints allows the crossed leg to be parallel to the floor your pelvis doesn't have to tilt as much, but you're still creating a challenge for vulnerable sciatic nerves.)

When your pelvis tilts, it draws your spine into temporary scoliosis (spine curves sideways right or left):

Your lumbar vertebrae in your lower spine curve sideways following your pelvis, and

Your vertebrae in your upper spine curve sideways in the opposite direction so that your head can remain upright.

Habitually sitting with the same leg crossed for long periods of time can irritate your sciatic nerves (and also cause blood circulation problems in your legs). Remember, part of the sciatic nerve network passes through the back of each knee.

Videotape is available from the Feldenkrais Guild office, which shows Moshe Feldenkrais being interviewed on TV. He was close to 80 years old, overweight, sitting in a thickly upholstered chair, and had a past history of very painful knees. In spite of all that, he demonstrated how he could stand up smoothly and quickly—because he had been sitting in acture with his feet solid on the floor.

Foot Placement Is Important While Sitting

When you sit, the placement of your feet influences how hard the muscles in your back must work to keep you upright.

Let's experiment so you can discover if this statement is true.

1 Sit forward enough on your chair so that your back (from your shoulders down through the back of your pelvis) is not touching the back of the chair.

2. Place your feet flat on the floor a comfortable distance apart, and bring yourself into your most comfortable posture.

3. Now, move your feet into a position where they are not flat on the floor. (For example, cross your ankles.)

   Did the change of foot position take you into a little bit of a slouch?

   If you were able to maintain your posture, did your back muscles have to work harder than when your feet were flat on the floor?

4. To verify if your foot position affects how hard your back must work to maintain your posture, slowly alternate between having your feet flat on the floor and not having one foot make firm contact with the floor.

Foot Placement Is Important When Standing

The position of your feet influences the position of your pelvis, and consequently, the comfort of your sciatic nerves as they thread from your lower lumbar vertebrae, through the back of your pelvis, and down your legs.

Standing with feet wide apart (military stance) tends to hyperextend knees. When your knees hyperextend, the knee joints actually bend backward beyond neutral. That's not healthful for either your knees or sensitive sciatic nerves.

If you stand with your feet wide apart and your knees hyperextended, your pelvis will either --

   Tilt so that your coccyx tucks under (eliminating your lumbar curve), or

   Tilt the opposite way (exaggerating your lumbar curve)

A more healthful option

Standing with one foot a little bit forward and one foot a little bit backward –

Encourages your pelvis to position your spine so that your lumbar curve is healthfully in place.

Enables you to shift your weight a bit forward or backward to help your back and legs be comfortable.

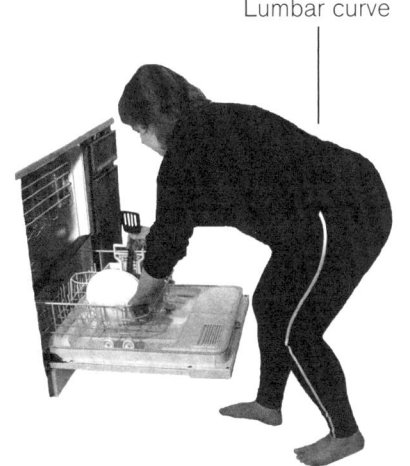

Lumbar curve

Foot Placement When Bending Over

Your back and sciatic nerves will be more comfortable any time you have to bend over if you place one foot back a little to help you maintain a lumbar curve. You want to lengthen your spine, not round it into a slouch. You need your coccyx (tail bone) released and your sternum (breastbone) facing forward, not downward. This is true *every time* you bend over—even if just bending over a little bit—washing your face, making the bed, adjusting the TV, etc.

Therapy While You Sleep

No mattress—no matter how firm—can keep your whole spine absolutely straight. To keep your spine "straight" you'd have to do the work, and that muscular tightening would make you less comfortable, not more comfortable. (Don't do it!) Hopefully, after you fell asleep, your body would have the wisdom to let some of that excessive muscle tension go.

When you relax while lying on your side, your spine gives in to gravity, curving a bit toward the ground. The softer the surface, the bigger the curve, but even when you lie on a hard floor, gravity draws your spine into a curve. Instead of tensing to try to keep your spine straight, use this gravity-induced curve for self-therapy.

The following therapeutic lesson utilizes gravity and your breathing to gently and subtly undulate your spine, thus improving circulation through your back and down through your legs.

Equipment needed: Two pillows, one for under your head, one for your legs, and a comfortable place to lie down

1 Lie on whichever side is the most comfortable for you.

2 Bend your knees to the degree that's comfortable for you. Then place a pillow between your legs *from your knees down to your toes.*

Note: Be sure that your bottom shoulder is under, not on top of, the pillow. You just want to support your neck without creating more of a challenge for your spine.

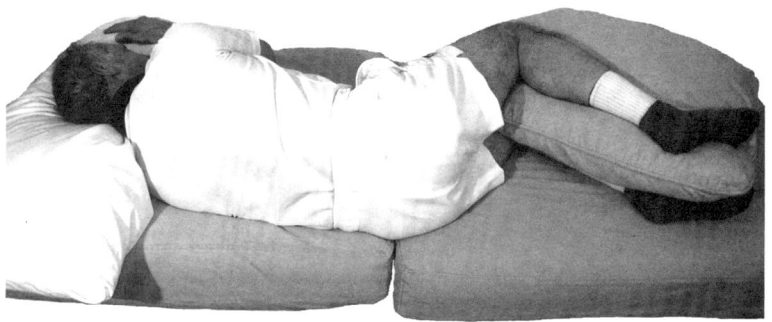

3 For a brief moment, try to keep your spine as straight as a stick, parallel to the floor.

> Sense if that makes your back less, instead of more, comfortable. Can you breathe very easily when you do that?

> Let that go!

4 Exaggerate your exhalation several times, allowing your inhalation to just naturally follow.

> As you exhale, the side of your rib basket nearest the ceiling can fold or "cave-in." Because your spine connects to your ribs, this subtly relaxes your spine a bit more toward the floor in a gentle curve.

> As you inhale, that upper side of your rib basket stops "caving in" and lifts your spine.

Reorganize Skeletally

It's the gentle undulation of the whole length of your spine, down into the deeper curve and back up, that's therapeutic—so don't fight it by tensing or guarding any part of your body. Don't even tense your jaw!

5   Each time you inhale allow your back to widen. Your lungs are like balloons. They don't just expand forward but also out to the sides and into your back.

   This relaxes your whole back all the way down through your pelvis, where your sciatic nerves thread to reach each leg.

   You will eventually find that your lower back can expand a bit with each inhalation. When you really relax you may even feel movement under your coccyx.

Note: If you choose to sleep on your back, place a folded pillow under your knees and make sure the pillow under your head is not too high.

Your Personal Progress Notes

4 Gentle Exercises to Reduce Pain

This chapter teaches you a variety of ways to be your own therapist whether you're at home, in the office, or traveling. These techniques will help you calm overactive muscles and sciatica pain.

Sitting Inch Worm

Many people with chronic lower back and leg pain tense both the front and the back of their bodies excessively. Contracting or tensing a muscle shortens it.

This exercise allows the muscles along both the front and the back of your spine to lengthen and relax.

1. Sit toward the edge of your bed, or on a chair, with your feet flat on the ground and your hands resting on your thighs.

2. Move your feet a little bit farther apart than usual and allow the same amount of space between your knees as between your feet.

3. Make sure your pelvis is supporting your spine (page 14 Posture From The Bottom Up) so that your sternum (breastbone) and your face are looking straight forward.

4. Without slouching, bend forward through your femoral (hip) joints.

    As you bend forward allow your coccyx (tail bone) to release— i.e. you're still sitting on the chair, but your coccyx no longer makes contact with the chair.

    As you bend forward allow your abdominal muscles to lengthen, not contract, so that your sternum can remain facing forward, not down toward the floor.

5   To return to your original upright position:

   ➢ Sink your sternum a little bit so it tilts toward your knees—as you sink your sternum, your spine will round into a little bit of a slouch, your head will sink forward, and your iliac crests (top of your hip bones) will tilt backward a bit.

   ➢ Then, reposition your pelvis so that your iliac crests are facing toward the ceiling (see page 14) and the vertebrae of your spine can stack up like "building blocks" from the bottom up.

   ➢ The neck end of your spine and your head will passively be the last to come up.

6   Slowly alternate between #4 (bend forward through your hip joints) and #5 (stack your spine like building blocks from the bottom up).

Standing Inch Worm

Excessively contracting the muscles in either the front of your body or along your spine pulls the vertebrae in your spine closer together and squishes the discs between them. This exercise opens and relaxes around your discs, and all the areas through which your sciatica nerves thread.

Allow your whole spine to participate, from the tip end of your coccyx to the top of your neck. Also allow your abdominal muscles to lengthen instead of contract.

Equipment needed: A sink, countertop, or tabletop

1   Rest your fingertips on the edge of a solid surface.

2   Stand with your feet parallel a comfortable distance apart, close enough to the countertop that your elbows are slightly bent while your hands rest on the edge.

3   "Accordion pleat," i.e. fold through your hip joints so that your coccyx (tailbone) releases backward and your knees bend a bit, as if you were about to sit down.

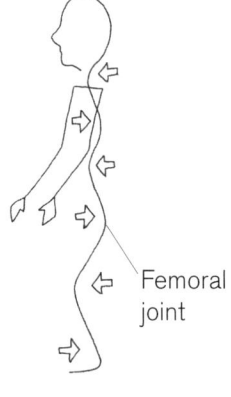
Femoral joint

Gentle Exercises to Reduce Pain   **25**

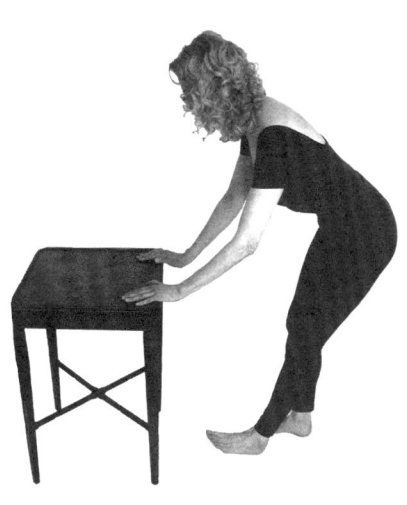

4. Slide one foot directly back until the toes of that foot are parallel to the heel of your other foot.

5. With your fingertips still resting on the countertop, draw your coccyx (tailbone) backward until your torso tilts forward a bit and the toes of your front foot passively release from the floor.

   The toes of your front foot pop off of the ground because your leg connects to and follows your pelvis, which is moving backward. Let your front foot relax and just rock a bit on the heel which remains in contact with the ground.

Important: Be sure you allow your coccyx to be released backward, not tucked. The backward movement of your coccyx lengthens and relaxes your spine because your spine is a continuum that includes your sacrum (the center back of your pelvis) and your coccyx.

6. With your fingertips still resting on the countertop, let your sacrum move forward—but not tuck under—until the toes of your front foot return to the ground, your head moves upward, and the heel of your back foot leaves the ground.

   This forward movement of your pelvis gently pushes your spine upward. Your chest moves forward and upward because your ribs wrap around from your spine to your sternum (breastbone).

   Allow the *front* and the *back* of your spine to lengthen up to the top of your neck. (Don't arch your neck.)

   Allow your lower back to gently regain its natural lumbar curve. This is the opposite of flattening your lower back.

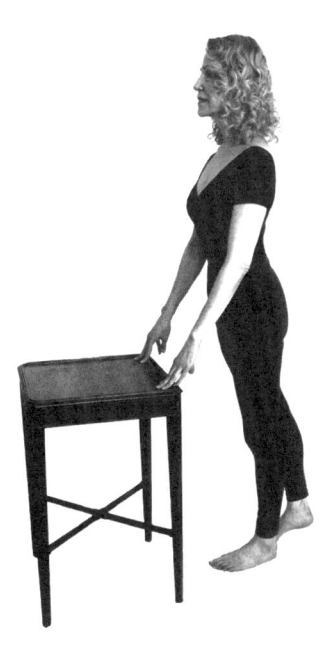

7. With your face looking forward throughout, *slowly and gently*:

   ➢ Fold a bit through your hip joints and knees with your coccyx released (not tucked) as if you were about to sit down

   ➢ Lengthen the back (and the front) of your spine as your coccyx leads backward

   ➢ Lengthen the front (and the back) of your spine as your sacrum moves forward (without tucking your coccyx) so you reach your full height

Relax Around Your Sciatic Nerves

This technique has been a "break through" to comfort for many of my clients. It encourages breathing more fully to give one's whole back a relaxing massage from the inside out.

Equipment needed: Padding for under your knees and lower legs, and a padded surface as high as your femoral joints when you are kneeling (possibilities include a coffee table padded with a pillow, or your bed if you have padding to put under your knees and lower legs, firm and high enough to bring your femoral joints up to the edge of the bed)

Note: The femoral joint is the ball-and-socket joint where your legs connect to your pelvis.

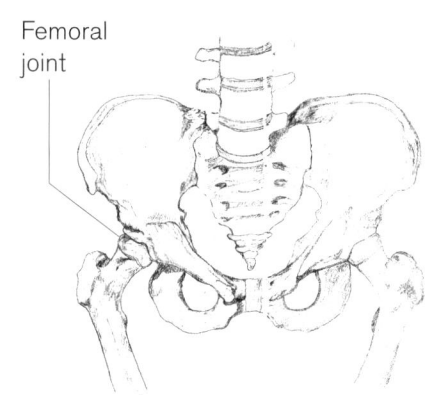

Femoral joint

1. Kneel near the edge of the padded surface, your knees a comfortable distance apart. Make sure your knees and lower legs are on padding thick enough for comfort.

2. Bend through your femoral joints. Allow your body to relax on the padded surface from your femoral joints to the top of your head.

3. Let your head rest whatever way is most comfortable.

4. Let your arms relax, with one hand resting near your face and the other arm resting down along your side.

5. Breathe with the awareness that your lungs are like balloons that can expand backward and out to the sides as well as forward. Your whole back can respond.

    Each time you inhale, allow your back to widen and your spine to lengthen in a relaxed way.

    Each time you exhale, think "Relax."

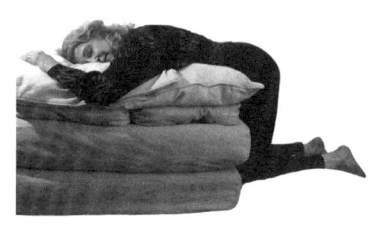

Note: This widening and lengthening of your back can happen with every breath you take, even when you are sitting or standing.

6. Allow your sacrum and coccyx to be lifted **passively** with each inhalation. As your rib basket responds to your breath, your whole spine can respond since your spine passes through the back of your rib basket and on down through your sacrum to the tip end of your coccyx.

Knee To Chest

This technique is frequently taught with the instruction to keep your back pinned to the surface. However, if you allow your pelvis (instead of your arms) to gently move your knee toward and away from your chest, the exercise becomes even more effective therapy for your back and your legs.

Important! Don't go to the maximum. If you can bring your knee to within 12 inches of your chest, only bring it to within 15 or 16 inches.

Equipment needed: a padded surface big enough for you to lie down with your knees bent (can be your bed)

1. Lie on your back on a padded surface.

2. Bend your knees and place your feet a comfortable distance apart. Relax your arms down by your sides.

3. Assess which side of your lower back is more comfortable. (Even if your whole back is tender, one side may be slightly less tense.)

4. With both knees bent, feet flat on the ground, and arms relaxed by your sides, draw **the knee on your more comfortable side** toward your chest.

    You do this without your arms pulling your leg!

5. **Tilt your pelvis to bring your knee toward your chest.** Your coccyx will rise a bit toward the ceiling and your lumbar vertebrae will gently press into the ground.

    The tilt of your pelvis acts as a fulcrum, bringing your knee toward your chest. This tilt also opens and relaxes the area through which your sciatic nerves pass to reach each leg.

6. Allow your pelvis to relax to its original position as you return your raised foot to the ground.

Note: If you keep your lower back pinned to the ground, you cannot use your pelvis as a fulcrum.

7   With both knees bent *and your first foot remaining in solid contact with the ground*, tilt your pelvis to bring your other knee toward your chest, allowing that side of your back to relax into the ground.

8   **Slowly and gently**, tilt your pelvis to bring one knee and then the other toward your chest.

   Each foot will take its turn alternately leaving the ground and then returning to the ground.

   Between pelvic tilts both feet will be flat on the ground.

9   Relax your rib basket so that your whole spine can move— including your neck!

   Each time your pelvis tilts to bring a knee toward your chest, allow your whole spine to be gently pushed in the direction of the top of your head so that your chin tilts away from your chest.

   Each time your pelvis settles into the ground to bring your foot down, allow your whole spine to be gently pulled by your pelvis in the direction of your feet so that the back of your neck lengthens and your chin is drawn toward your chest.

Movement through your neck and head is a good indication you are doing therapy for your whole spine as you do this exercise.

Gentle Exercises to Reduce Pain

➢ Let your chin be pushed away from your chest each time your spine is nudged in the direction of the top of your head as your knee goes toward your chest.

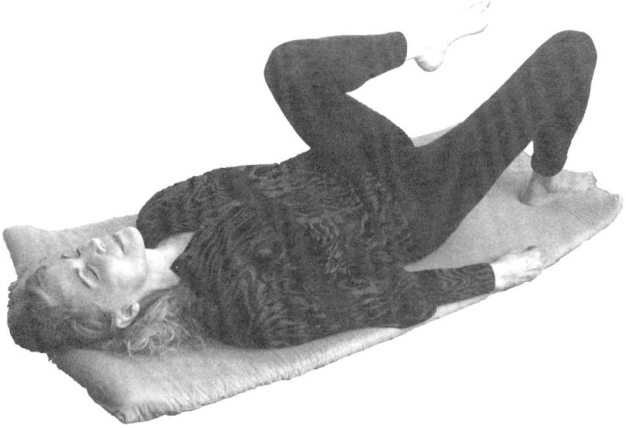

➢ Allow your chin to be drawn toward your chest each time your pelvis returns your foot to the ground.

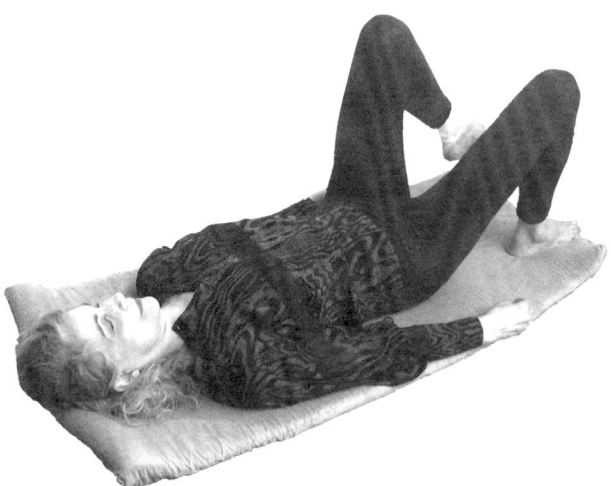

10 As you rest, notice if your lower back and your legs are more comfortable!

Less Is More

You can soothe your sciatic nerve network by rubbing it gently with a rolled up sock or foam rubber ball similar to a NERF® Ball. A tennis ball, even if it has lost its bounce, is too hard. You're going to roll this ball along the path of your sciatic nerve network.

What follows are two versions of the technique.

Less Is Better Than More, Version I

This position of this exercise is the same as the exercise in "Relax Around Your Sciatic Nerves," on page 26.

Equipment needed: a rolled up sock or very soft foam rubber ball similar to a NERF® Ball, and a padded surface as high as your femoral joints when you are kneeling (possibilities include a coffee table padded with a pillow, or your bed if you have padding to put under your knees and lower legs, firm and high enough to bring your femoral joints up to the edge of the bed).

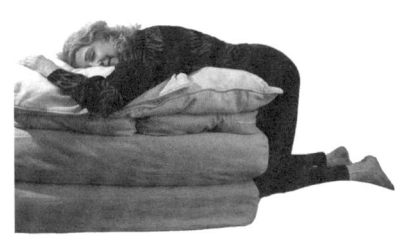

1. Kneel near the edge of a padded surface. Make sure your lower legs and feet are on padding thick enough for comfort.

2. Bend through your femoral joints. Allow your body to relax on the padded surface from your femoral joints to the top of your head. Turn your head to one side.

3. Let your arms relax, with one hand resting near your face and the other arm resting down along your side. Have the soft ball in the hand of the arm that is resting down along your side.

4. *With your lower body relaxed*, roll the soft ball wherever you can comfortably reach. Possibilities include –

    ➢ Around the lumbar vertebrae in your lower back

    ➢ Over your sacrum

    ➢ Down the back of your thigh

5. Allow your back to respond to your breath! This should not be hard work. If it starts to feel that way—lighten your touch and your effort.

Less Is Better Than More, Version 2

This version is very similar to the exercise in Knee to Chest, which begins on page 27.

If any of these exercises start to feel like hard work in any way, reduce your effort to the point that you don't interfere with your breathing

Equipment needed: A rolled up sock or very soft foam rubber ball similar to a NERF® Ball and a padded surface, big enough for you to lie down with your knees bent

1. Lie on your back with your knees bent and your feet a comfortable distance apart. Hold a soft ball in one hand.

2. Assess which side of your lower back is more comfortable and use the leg on that side first. (Even if your whole back is tender, one side may be slightly less tense.)

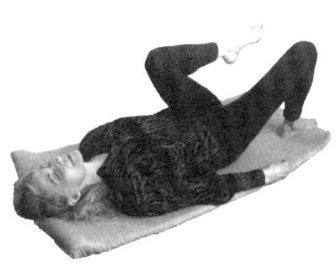

3. With both knees bent, feet flat on the ground, and your arms relaxed by your sides, let your pelvis tilt backward to draw your most comfortable-side knee toward your chest.

4. Remaining as relaxed as possible, roll the soft ball from your buttocks up the back of your thigh to the back of your knee several times.

Note: Roll the ball so gently it remains spherical, not flattened.

5. Allow your rib basket to be relaxed and pliable so that you can reach comfortably to roll the soft ball down the front of your lower leg on the outside edge of your shin bone several times.

6. Roll the soft ball up the back of your thigh and down the front of your leg several times, making a circle.

7. Now, gently repeat Steps 3, 4, 5, and 6 with your other leg.

Cradle Your Leg

This technique uses a sling to encourage your lower back, back of your pelvis, your hip joint, and your leg to let go of excess muscular tension so that your network of nerves can calm down. You can do the exercise alone or with the assistance of a friend.

Stop and rest anytime you feel this is uncomfortable work. It should be pleasurable therapy.

Equipment needed: pillowcase or towel long enough to use as a sling for your leg, and a padded surface on which to lie

1 Lie on your back on your bed or on a padded floor with both knees bent and both feet flat on the ground, a comfortable distance apart.

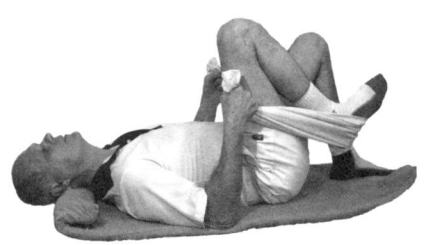

2 Bring the knee on your more comfortable side toward your chest—by tilting your pelvis so that your lower back presses into the ground.

3 Use the pillowcase or towel as a sling for your heel, holding the ends of the material with your hands.

4 Allow your foot to be supported in the air by the sling so that your leg can relax and give in to gravity.

> Allow your elbows to rest on the ground so your arms and shoulders can relax as much as possible.
>
> Stay this way until you feel that your leg can truly allow its weight to be supported by the sling.
>
> Allow your toes to relax so you don't create any tension in the leg. Allow your jaw to relax.

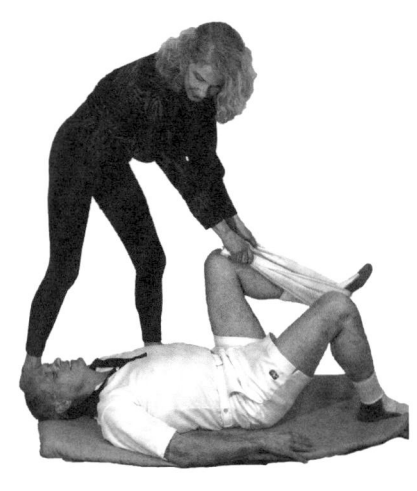

Note: If someone is available to help you, that person can stand near your upper body, holding and moving the sling for you.

Gentle Exercises to Reduce Pain

5   Without changing your grip on the sling, move your hands in the direction of the supported foot—just enough so that the sling and your foot travel a little bit toward the floor. Then, gently pull the sling and your foot toward you again.

You'll get faster results if your leg remains passive.

Do this forward and back movement several times to encourage your leg and hip joint to relax.

If you sense that your leg is doing the work for you, go back to Step 4 until your leg can allow itself to be moved passively.

6   Each time the sling and your foot are gently pulled toward you, allow your pelvis to passively tilt.

7   Slide the sling up from your heel to support the ball of your foot.

8   As in Step 5 allow the foot in the sling to be lowered a bit and then drawn back toward your body to cue your leg and hip joint to relax.

9   Let this foot return all the way to the floor and slide the sling out from underneath.

10 As you rest, sense any difference in how your back and leg feel after this treatment.

11 Now gently and slowly do all of the above with your other leg.

Your Personal Progress Notes

5 Constructive Fidgeting

Gentle movement is the path out of pain! Many people think that first nudge of pain yells, "Don't move or you'll cause more pain!" Actually, the opposite is true.

Take an ergonomically ideal office environment and add people with no pre-existing physical problems and long hours spent working at computers. Some of these people will experience pain while others will not. What's the difference?

Often the difference is that people who remain pain free don't stay "stock still." It's a combination of awareness and what one might call "healthful restlessness."

Our bodies were meant to move! It takes inhibition to keep us from moving. As we sleep, hormones provide that inhibition. When we're awake, we often inhibit through muscular tension.

The activities in this chapter are some examples of "constructive fidgeting" techniques that you can use to prevent or eliminate pain while sitting at your desk or in the theater. You can even use them while sitting with your seatbelt buckled in a car or on an airplane.

Key Points To Remember

- ➢ We need to remind ourselves that we were not designed to stay "stock still" for more than just a brief period of time.

- ➢ Your movement can be a massage for you—from the inside out—to relax areas that are starting to become uncomfortable.

- ➢ Sometimes we need to give ourselves permission to move.

- ➢ To be an effective therapist for yourself, move slowly and gently.

Intentional Slouching as a Technique

Note: This constructive fidgeting technique is not intended to suggest that it's a good idea to remain in a slouch. It's not in your best interest to remain for a long time with the top of your sacrum (center back of your pelvis) tilted backward right at its junction with your bottom lumbar vertebra (disc between L5 S1).

"Intentional" is the key word here. When you sense that you may be slouching, consciously sink into a bit more of a slouch so that you can then bring yourself out of the slouch in the most healthful way.

Intentional, **brief**, slouching can wake up your mind while it renews flexibility in your back. In some grade schools where *Feldenkrais®* is used for students and teachers, techniques like Intentional Slouching are called "*alertness breaks*."

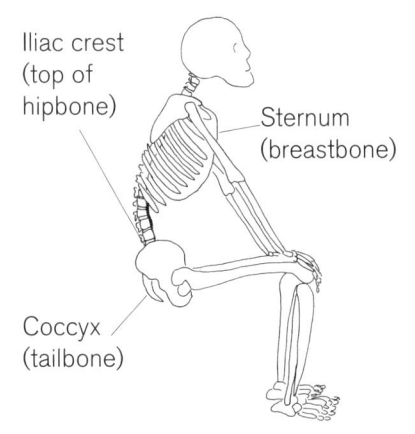

Equipment needed: ideally a firm chair, but you can do this wherever you happen to be sitting—at your desk, in your car, on an airplane, or at the theater.

1 Sink your chest to make your upper back round backward.

   To be skeletally specific: Your ribs wrap around to connect your sternum and your spine. So when your sternum sinks inward and downward, your ribs round your spine backward into a slouch.

2 Lift your chest forward and up.

   As your sternum lifts forward and up, your ribs lead your upper spine forward and up so that your upper back is less rounded.

3 Alternate between sinking and lifting your chest.

   Allow your mid-and-lower spine to follow your upper spine as it's led by the sinking and lifting of your ribs and sternum.

   Each time your sternum lifts, allow your entire spine (from the tip end of your tailbone to the top of your neck) to respond.

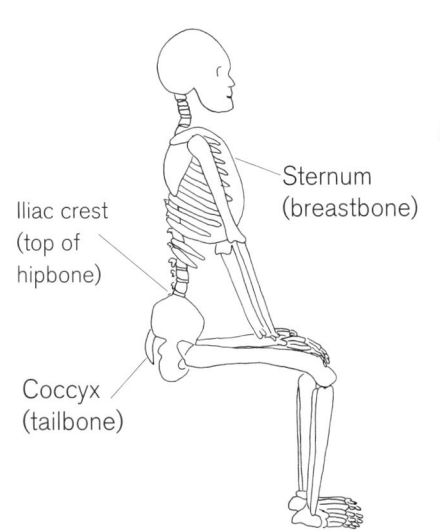

4   Continue alternating between sinking and lifting your chest.

> As you sink your sternum and round your back, notice that your iliac crests (the tops of your hip bones) tilt backward.

> As you lift your sternum and your spine moves forward and up, notice that your iliac crests move forward a bit.

So far you've let your sternum lead the process. This is a good way to begin when your lower back is very painful. Now, let your pelvis take you into more upright posture after each time your sternum sinks you into a slouch.

5   The next time your sternum is sunken and your back is rounded, roll your iliac crests (top of your hip bones) forward in the direction of the ceiling (page 14). Your pelvis has now rearranged your spine to lift your ribs and sternum. You are no longer sitting on your coccyx.

6   Gently alternate between sinking your sternum to round your spine, then repositioning your iliac crests so that your sternum goes forward and up and you're not leaning on your coccyx.

Gentle Side-Folding Through Your Ribs

Side-folding through your ribs and upper spine helps overactive muscles relax. As your upper spine becomes more flexible your lower spine will free up and your whole back will become more comfortable.

When you focus skeletally, instead of muscularly, your nervous system activates *only* the muscles necessary for that particular movement. As you do this exercise think skeletally!

1   Sit with your pelvis supporting your spine (page14) and your feet flat on the floor a comfortable distance apart.

2   Gently collapse one side of your rib basket, as if you wanted to reach down sideways to pick something up.

> **Important!** Don't just bend through the waist. Instead, make sure that you bend and fold through your mid and upper rib basket (all the way up under your arm).

3. Slowly alternate sinking to one side and then the other.

   Exhale as you collapse one side of your rib basket

   Inhale as you come up to center.

   As one side of your spine folds, the other side opens.

4. Try this side-folding of your ribs while standing, with your feet parallel and with a slight fold through your hip joints and knees.

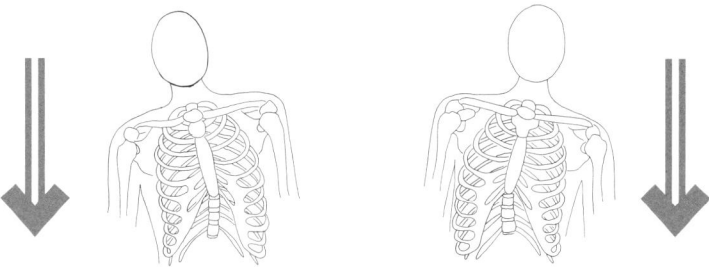

Gentle Spine Stretches

The discs between the vertebrae in your spine act as cushions. You compact those discs when you habitually flatten your back or you habitually slouch. This exercise allows those discs to plump up again.

What follows are two versions of the technique, one while sitting and the other while standing.

Sitting, Gentle Spine Stretch

This example of constructive fidgeting allows one side of your spine and then the other to lengthen and stretch, counteracting the effects of gravity.

Equipment needed: Ideally a firm chair, but you can do this wherever you happen to be sitting—at your desk, on an airplane, or in a theater.

1. Determine which side of your body is more comfortable—your "1st side."

Constructive Fidgeting

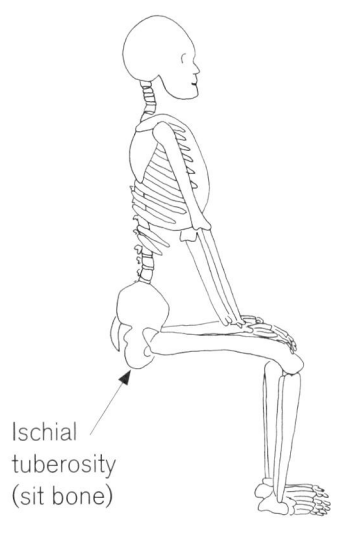

Ischial tuberosity (sit bone)

2. Shift your weight over your "1st side" ischial tuberosity ("sit bone") and allow that side of your spine and rib basket to stretch open. Then return to your neutral starting position.

3. Now slowly shift your weight onto the "sit bone" on your 2nd side so that the 2nd side of your spine can lengthen in a gentle stretch all the way up under your ear.

4. Each time one side of your spine stretches open (lengthens), allow your head and shoulders to be passively tilted toward the other side.

> As one side of your spine opens, the other side folds. As one side of your spine lengthens, the other side shortens into a curve.

> As one side of your rib basket opens, the ribs on your other side simultaneously fold.

> As you shift your weight onto one "sit bone," your other one rises a little bit.

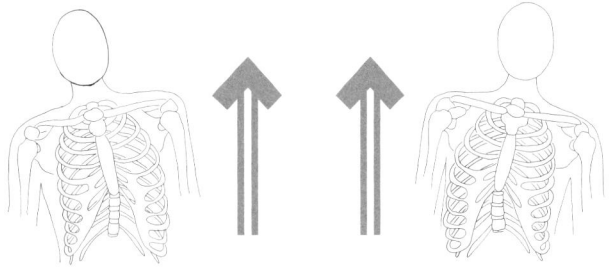

5. Shift side to side, slowly enough to allow one side of your rib basket to open and your spine to lengthen; and then the other side of your rib basket to open and spine to lengthen.

Standing, Gentle Spine Stretch

This wonderful exercise is subtle enough you can do it wherever you want to and whenever you want to. It's especially good to get this lengthening of your spine at the end of the day if it feels like gravity has compacted your spine.

1. Stand with your feet a comfortable distance apart, your weight evenly supported by both feet.

If you're at all unsure about your balance, let your fingertips rest on a countertop or the back of a chair. Just don't grip tightly.

2. Determine which side of your body is more comfortable. For this exercise, also, your more comfortable side is your "1st side."

3. Shift your weight over your "1st side" foot. Let it solidly support you.

The heel of the other foot will leave the ground but the front half of that foot remains in contact with the ground as you shift your weight away from it.

4. As your 1st-side foot presses into the ground, let that side of your spine stretch all the way up through the side of your neck.

Allow the ribs on your 1st side to stretch open each time that side of your spine gently stretches.

Allow your shoulders to relax so they passively "seesaw" during this stretch.

5. Shift your weight over the foot on your 2nd side and gently allow all of the above in #3 and #4 to accompany the stretch of that second side.

6. Slowly shift your weight onto one foot and then the other.

As your weight shifts onto your right foot, let the right side of your spine "get tall."

As your weight shifts to your left, let the left side of your spine "get tall."

Side-to-Side Rib Wiggle

You can improve your comfort, flexibility, and circulation by gently moving your ribs side-to-side. This "snakes" your spine all the way up through your neck and all the way down through the back of your pelvis.

Equipment needed: Ideally a firm chair, but you can do this wherever you happen to be sitting—at your desk, in your car, or at the theater.

Constructive Fidgeting 41

1. Gently shift your weight onto one "sit" bone and then onto the other—*as* in "Sitting Gentle Spine Stretch," but with smaller, quicker movements, like Jell-O® jiggling.

2. As you shift back and forth, notice that your ribs –

    ➤ Travel sideways to follow your pelvis, and

    ➤ Fold on the side opposite the move's direction

    As you shift your weight onto your right sit bone, the right side of your rib basket opens and the left side folds.

    As you shift your weight onto your left sit bone, the left side of your rib basket opens and the right side folds.

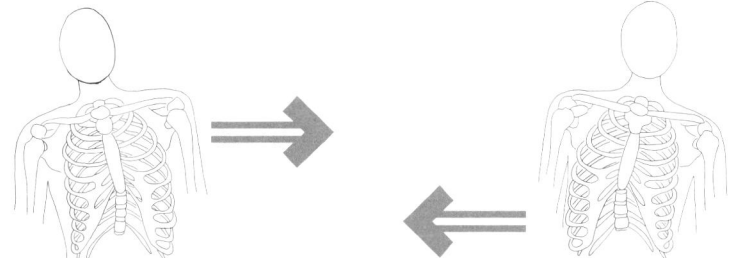

3. Begin to lead the side-to-side motion with your ribs instead of with your pelvis.

    Allow your whole spine to follow your rib basket so that your pelvis tilts a little bit to one side and then the other.

    Don't prevent the neck-end of your spine from participating. Allow the top of your head to passively tilt back and forth, away from the side that is stretching.

Note: You can do the Side-to-Side Rib Wiggle while sitting, standing, or lying on your back. This is a wonderful way to (literally) shake off stress.

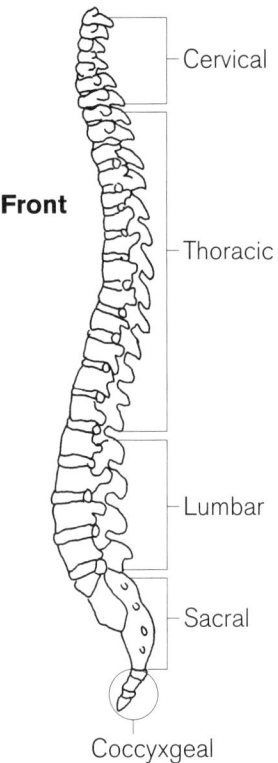

Shake off your stress

When you feel stressed, your chest probably stiffens and your breathing may minimize—like a deer frozen in front of a car's headlights. This is the formula that turns your potentially pliable rib "basket" into a rib "cage."

Because your ribs connect to your thoracic vertebrae, when your chest stiffens and your rib basket becomes a rib "cage" you trap the thoracic vertebrae of your spine. Why is this significant? That's trapping *half* your total movable vertebrae!

Human beings have 24 movable vertebrae: 7 cervical (neck), 12 thoracic (rib), and 5 lumbar (lower back). The sacral and coccyxgeal vertebrae are fused. When you trap the thoracic (rib) section of your spine—as if those 12 individual bones were a single "backbone"—the 7 cervical vertebrae above and the 5 lumbar vertebrae below sustain extra wear and tear.

By regaining the flexibility of your rib basket, you can reduce vulnerability in your lower back. Regaining flexibility through your rib basket and spine counteracts the muscle contraction and nerve impingement that can cause sciatic nerve pain.

6 More Self-Help Techniques

The intention of this chapter is to widen your menu of ways to reverse and prevent sciatic nerve pain. All these exercises are indexed at the end of the book so that, on any given day, you can choose several from the menu.

Walk Backward

Walking backward can encourage over-active muscles in your back to relax. Walking backward also encourages "accordion pleating" so that your healthful lumbar curve returns and your skeleton is organized for comfort and efficiency.

For information about:

➤ "Accordion pleating," see page 16

➤ Sciatic nerve path, see Chapter 2, beginning on page 7

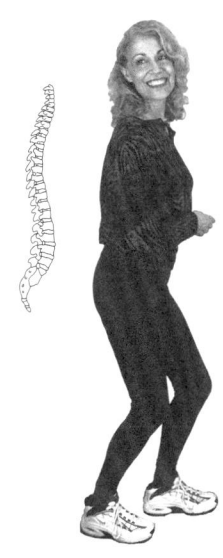

1. Lead with your sacrum (sacral vertebrae in center back of your pelvis), not with your feet.

    This encourages your coccyx to un-tuck. If you have been habitually tucking your coccyx under you, this might feel a little unusual. However, it's just what your need to relieve sciatic pain.

2. Let your shoulders, arms, and jaw relax.

3. Allow your abdominal muscles to lengthen, instead of contract, so that the front of you is not bent over. This enables your head to be vertically over your body without tensing your neck.

You only need to walk backward a few steps to get some relief, so you can do this subtly while in a museum or at the mall. Just—please—make sure there's nothing behind you to trip over!

Cat/Camel with Skeletal Awareness

There is a yoga expression:

"You are as young as your spine is supple."

The traditional "cat/camel" yoga exercise to help flexibility becomes even more effective when you add Feldenkrais® and skeletal awareness. This will help you open and relax areas through which the sciatic nerves pass.

Optional equipment: padding under your knees and hands such as exercise mat, garden kneeling pads, pillows, or shoulder pads discarded from blouses or jackets. (You could do this exercise on your bed.)

1. Move on to your hands and knees, making sure that –

    ➢ Your hands are shoulders' width apart

    ➢ Your knees are under your hips

    ➢ Your feet are as widely placed as your knees

2. Round your back like an angry cat, but don't go to your maximum.

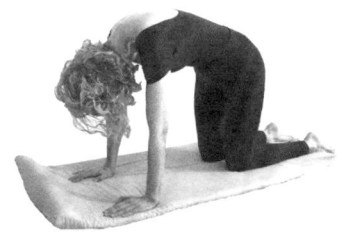

    Notice that, as your spine rounds upward like a hill, your coccyx (tail bone) tucks under you, your lumbar curve disappears, and your head is drawn toward your chest.

    This opens and lengthens the back of your spine and all the areas through which your sciatic nerves pass, **however...**

    This is a slouch, so just stay there briefly!

3. Now, allow your back to relax in neutral (like a table instead of a swayback camel).

    Note: This is **not** a push-up exercise; but rather a rounding and un-rounding of your spine. Your arms remain straight.

    Notice that your healthful lumbar curve returns as you un-tuck your coccyx and your upper back flattens instead of rounds.

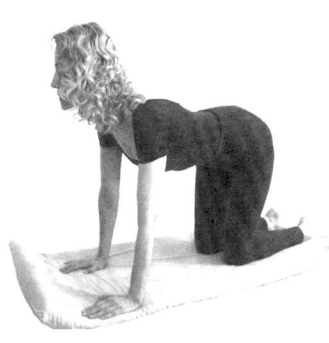

4. Allow your sternum (breastbone), to move forward and up, lengthening the front of your body and passively lifting your head. This is the position in which babies crawl.

> When your sternum sinks you into a slouch, the front of your spine curls and the back of your spine lengthens. However, as your sternum lifts, the front of you lengthens and your lower back curves into a gentle lumbar curve.

Note: If you've been chronically guarding your back, you may not be able to lengthen the front of your body very much at all right now. Be gentle with yourself. That will improve as you repeat this exercise over time.

Alternate between:

- ➢ Caving in your chest, which rounds your spine into a hill/slouch, and
- ➢ Moving your sternum forward/upward and releasing your coccyx, which allows your spine to have a lumbar curve.

Remember: Your spine is a continuum all the way from the top of your neck down through the center back of your pelvis (sacrum) to the tip end of your coccyx (tail bone).

Free Your Upper Back/Help Your Lower Back

If your lower back and pelvis seem stuck in pain, you can regain comfort and flexibility by mobilizing your upper spine!

Although the position of this exercise may, at first, seem a bit awkward, the benefits can be profound. This exercise gently opens and relaxes all of the areas through which the sciatic nerve network passes.

Equipment needed: padded floor (thick carpet, thick blanket, or exercise mat), and a book or gardening kneeling pad

1. Kneel on your knees and elbows (like a sphinx). Position your lower legs, from your knees to your toes, parallel on the ground; your lower arms, from your elbows to your fingertips, parallel on the ground.

2. Place your forehead between your fingertips on the ground (or on a book or gardening kneeling pad).

3. With your head remaining in contact with "the ground" and your lower legs and lower arms relaxed into the ground, move your pelvis in the direction of your head.

   As your pelvis moves forward, allow your spine to round into a hill, all the way up through your neck.

   This rolls your head a little bit more toward the top of your skull since your spine is the connecting link between your pelvis and head.

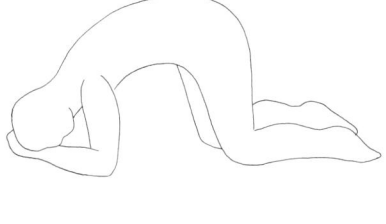

Important! Don't let your head lift from, or slide on, the ground—you just want it to be rolled by your pelvis in a relaxed way. If this is uncomfortable for your head, turn your palms up and let the weight of your head sink into your hands. Just make sure your shoulders can relax.

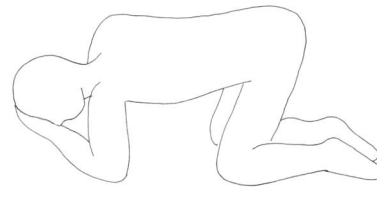

4. Now, with your head still making contact with the ground or the palms of your hands, move your pelvis away from your head. (If you've chosen to have your hands cradle your head, keep the back of your hands in contact with the ground so that your hands and head don't lift from the ground.)

   Allow this backward movement of your pelvis to:

   ➢ Roll your head so that your chin moves toward the ground, and

   ➢ Draw your spine out of the hill and into a gentle lumbar curve.

Remember: Your whole spine, including your neck, can follow your pelvis because your spine is a continuum that includes your sacrum (center back of your pelvis).

5   About eight times, **slowly** and gently alternate between:

> ➣ Moving your pelvis forward, which rounds the spine and rolls your head more toward the top of your skull, and
>
> ➣ Moving your pelvis backward, which draws your head more toward your nose and chin.

Remember: Allow your head to roll, not lift, so that you remain relaxed and your spine and sciatic nerves can benefit.

> ➣ The forward movement, when you roll toward the top of your head, is important for contrast
>
> ➣ However, it's the backward movement, when your head rolls toward your chin, that gives a healthful lengthening stretch to your spine—down to your coccyx (tailbone) and through the areas where your sciatic nerves thread.

6   As you continue slowly moving your pelvis forward and backward, allow your shoulders and neck to relax, enabling this movement to travel through your upper spine.

7   Notice the section of your spine that runs between your scapulae (shoulder blades) as you continue slowly moving your pelvis forward and backward. Mobilizing this area is key to helping relieve your sciatica.

> ➣ As your pelvis moves forward and your spine rounds into a hill, allow the section of your spine between your scapulae to rise as part of the hill.
>
> ➣ As your pelvis moves backward, drawing your spine into a gentle stretch and rolling your head more toward your nose, allow the section of spine between your scapulae to sink. This is the part of the exercise to gently emphasize.

8   As you rest, notice if this mobilization of your upper spine made your lower back more comfortable.

Roll to Iron Out Your Back

This technique helps relax the muscles through your back and your whole sciatic nerve network.

Equipment needed: A padded surface big enough to lie down on with your knees bent and your feet flat (could be your bed), referred to in this exercise as "the ground."

1. Lie on your back with your knees bent and your feet flat on "the ground."

2. Determine which side of your body is more comfortable. This is the "1st side" of your body.

3. Gently tilt your pelvis to draw the knee on the 1st side of your body toward your chest.

   Important! Don't go to the maximum. If you can draw your knee to within 12 inches of your chest, only draw it to within 18 inches.

   Allow the 1st side of your back to relax onto the surface with your foot off the surface.

4. Once you feel the relaxation on your first side, draw the knee on the 2nd side of your body toward your chest too.

   With both knees toward your chest, allow both sides of your back to relax and lengthen onto the surface with both feet off the surface.

5. With your back, shoulders, and neck relaxed, rest your hands on the top or sides of your knees, right hand in contact with your right knee, left hand with your left knee.

6. Gently roll side-to-side to "iron out" your back. Allow the neck end of your spine to follow so that your head is passively rolled.

7. Continue this motion until you feel you've rolled enough to relax your whole back, including the back of your pelvis. Then, allow first one foot, and then the other, to return to "the ground."

8   Gently wiggle through your ribs to appreciate the degree of comfort through the whole length of your spine, from the top of your neck down to your coccyx (tail bone).

Flexible Rib Basket/Flexible Spine

Many of you have been instructed not to rotate since you have a history of lower back difficulties. However, you must twist from time to time—to reach for something, to talk to someone behind you, to back the car out of the driveway, or for sports such as golf, tennis, baseball, and skiing.

Through the following lesson you'll learn to twist without jeopardizing your lower back—*allowing the twist to happen through your rib basket.*

Important: Someone who has never had lower back problems could eventually *create* lower back problems by keeping the rib basket like a "cage" restricting thoracic (rib) vertebrae from helping lumbar vertebrae to rotate. As a preventive measure, going in and out of asymmetry through your rib basket can help keep your back supple and less vulnerable.

Each thoracic (rib) vertebra has the ability to rotate up to 20 degrees while each lumbar vertebra can only rotate one degree. This lesson will help you return your rib "cage," to the rib "basket" nature intended, helping the flexibility of your thoracic vertebrae, the flexibility of your whole back.

Equipment needed: your bed or a padded surface big enough for you to lie down with your legs lengthened

1   Lie on your back and take a moment to sense which side of your body is more comfortable.

2   Bend your more-comfortable-side knee so that your foot is solidly on the ground. Your other leg remains straight and relaxed.

3   Tilt your bent knee a little bit inward toward your straight leg. Then return your bent knee to its upright ("neutral") position.

each time

4. Now tilt your bent knee again, but this time also let your pelvis roll a bit in the direction of your leg that's straight as your bent knee tilts inward and then returns to neutral.

> Now you're allowing both the "socket" (acetabulum in your pelvis) and the "ball" of your femur (thigh bone) to move together.
>
> Do this several times and notice if your hip joint and leg are more comfortable when you let your pelvis move.

Remember: Your sciatic nerves thread through the bottom of your femoral (hip) joint where your leg attaches to your pelvis.

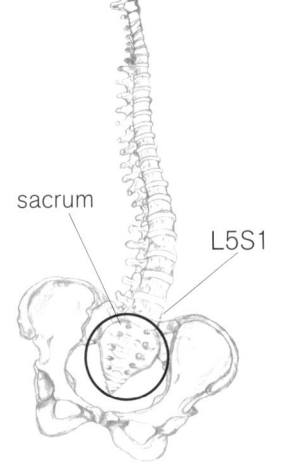

sacrum

L5S1

5. Notice if the straightened leg that is resting on the floor also rolls a little bit as your pelvis and bent knee roll.

> Both legs are ball-and-socketed to your pelvis. As your pelvis rolls, every part of your skeleton that is attached to it will move—if you allow it to.

6. Notice that your lower back wants to follow your pelvis. Allow that to happen.

> You don't have to make your lower back follow; you just have to get out of your own way. It actually takes *counterproductive* muscular effort to prevent your lower back from following your pelvis.

Important: Trying to "guard" (trying to prevent your lumbar vertebrae from following your pelvis) can create problems at L5 S1 where the lowest lumbar vertebrae meet the top of your sacrum. Remember your spine is a continuum that includes your sacrum so allow your whole spine to follow—including the vertebrae that have ribs attached.

More Self-Help Techniques

7. Allow your rib basket to become asymmetrical as you twist so that your upper spine can also be mobile.

   Allowing your ribs to mobilize your upper spine, helps your lower spine be less vulnerable and more comfortable.

8. Rest for a moment.

   Note: As you rest, think about how this isn't just an exercise for flexibility, but the path for returning to a pain-free life.

9. Once again, bend the knee on the more comfortable side of your body so that your foot makes solid contact with the ground. Rest your arms on the ground six or eight inches from the sides of your body.

10. Become aware of the triangular space between your right arm and the right side of your body and the triangular space between your left arm and the left side of your body.

11. Let your whole body, including your shoulders, relax as your pelvis rolls your bent knee inward and then back to neutral.

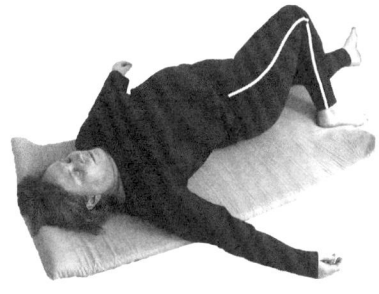

   If you allow your rib basket to respond *each time* your pelvis rolls your bent knee inward, the triangular space formed by the bent-knee side of your body and arm becomes larger.

   Your lowest ribs, on the bent-knee-side follow the roll of your pelvis first. It's a ripple-up effect with the ribs way up under your arm moving last.

   Then, as your pelvis and knee return to neutral, the ribs up under your arm on your bent-knee-side return to the ground first and the lowest ribs return to the ground last.

   This asymmetry of your rib basket indicates your shoulders and your rib basket are relaxed enough to allow your whole spine to follow the roll of your pelvis.

12 *Each time your pelvis rolls your knee inward*, allow your chin to be drawn a little bit downward toward your chest. This allows the back of your neck to lengthen so that your whole spine participates

13 As you rest, gently wiggle through your rib basket and allow your whole spine to respond. It's therapeutic!

14 When you are ready, repeat all the instructions with the other side of your body.

Notice that in all the exercises, the word "allow" is used frequently. Your body wants to be allowed to be freely mobile. As you allow your body to be more free, you will be more comfortable. You just need to learn how, and that's what this book is all about.

7 Moving through Your Day

The way to prevent sciatica from recurring is to be smart about the way you do everything—sitting, standing, working, exercising, and even relaxing. You don't have to curtail activities, but you do have to be conscious of how you move.

This chapter takes you through some of the activities in a typical day so that you can discover that:

➤ Making conscious decisions about how you move doesn't take more work—just more awareness.

➤ Making healthful choices based on your awareness of body position enables you to move through your day with more efficiency and more comfort.

Before You Get Out of Bed

While still lying in bed, you can gently wake up your spine by doing the following exercises which were taught in previous chapters. As you do the exercises, please remember:

➤ These are **gentle** "wake-ups." If any one becomes work, stop, wiggle through your ribs (page 41) and just breathe before you continue.

➤ Allow your head to rest on the bed throughout. Don't lift it.

➤ Allow your jaw to relax so that you don't create excessive muscular tension.

Wake-up exercise #1

1. Lie on your back with both knees bent so that your feet are flat on the bed. Allow your jaw to relax.

2. Have your pelvis alternately bring one knee a little bit toward your chest, and then the other. (Review "Knee to Chest" on pages 27-29.)

   Each time, tilt your pelvis so that your lower back gently presses into the bed. Let your whole spine, including your neck, respond.

Wake-up exercise 2

1. Lie on your back with both knees bent so that your feet are flat on the bed. Allow your jaw to relax.

2. Wiggle side-to-side through your rib basket to gently snake your spine. (Review page 41.)

Wake-up exercise 3

1. Lie on your back with your most-comfortable-side knee bent, the less-comfortable-side leg resting long on the bed with a pillow under that knee.

2. Have your pelvis gently roll from away from your bent-knee side and then relax back center. Allow the twist to happen up under your arms. (Review "Flexible Rib Basket/Flexible Spine" beginning on page 49.)

3. Allow your rib basket to be passively moved into and out of asymmetry so that the rolling of your spine, as it follows your pelvis, travels up through your neck.

Wake-up exercise 4

1. Lie on your back with both knees bent so that your feet are flat on the bed. Allow your jaw to relax.

2. Tilt your pelvis to bring one knee toward your chest. Then also bring the other knee toward your chest.

3. Let your hands hold your knees and roll a tiny bit side-to-side. (Review "Roll to Iron Out Your Back" on page 48.)

Get In and Out of Bed

The more you try to guard your lower back and use only your upper body to lie down or come up to sitting, the more apt you are to trigger lower body pain.

The way to keep your lower back **most comfortable,** as you move from a lying down position up to sitting, is to:

➢ Move from your pelvis.

➢ Let your pelvis be the fulcrum so that the weight of the lower half of your body can lift your upper body.

➢ Allow your lower back to be relaxed as possible so that excessive tension doesn't interfere.

➢ Allow your jaw, neck, and shoulder muscles to be relaxed so your upper body can passively follow, not interfere with, the movement of your pelvis.

Sitting Up From Lying Down

1 Lie on your back with your knees bent so that your feet are flat on the bed.

2 Bend both arms and rest them on your chest.

3 Keep both knees bent and touching each other so that the more comfortable leg can give support to the more vulnerable side of your body.

4 Have your pelvis roll you on to your side so that you're facing the edge of the bed where you will eventually sit.

> As you rest on your side, think about the line of direction you are going to travel as you come up to sitting. Don't move yet! Just think about moving.

If you begin by lifting the head end of your body up toward the ceiling, the muscles through your lower back and legs may clench.

Instead, spiral up. Let your pelvis roll you toward the edge of the bed. Then, when your bent legs go over the side of the bed, the weight of your lower body will pull the rest of your body upright. This is similar to those punch toys weighted on the bottom: push them over and they pop back up.

Now, let's put it all together:

5   With your upper body relaxed, let your pelvis roll to return you to lying on your back with your knees bent.

6   With knees still bent, let your pelvis roll you onto your side and allow your head to travel a bit over the edge of the bed so that you can see the floor.

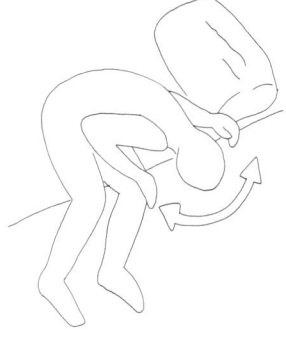

7   Let your bent legs go over the side of the bed and allow the weight of your lower body to **spiral** your upper body upright so that you are sitting on the edge of the bed with your feet on the floor. Your head is last to come up—not first.

The path you just traveled is reversible. To lie down on your bed, follow these steps.

8   Sit on the side of the bed and rest. As you rest, picture how you could reverse the path you just traveled so that you end up lying back down on the bed.

9   While still sitting on the edge of the bed, bend through your femoral joints (where your legs connect to your pelvis) so that your spine lengthens forward and your face is toward the floor.

> This is a good time to think about the very first experi-ment in the book (page 5) where you bent over in a sitting position with your spine lengthened instead of rounded.

10 Let your pelvis move the upper half of your body in a short practice arc that would return your head to the bed if you completed it. Then return through that same arc to sitting upright.

11 The next time let your pelvis move your body completing the arc.

> Allow your feet to leave the floor so your legs can follow your pelvis as your head settles on your pillow.

> If one leg is vulnerable support it with the other leg as you move through space.

12 Pause on your side where your pelvis deposited you with your knees bent. Then roll from your pelvis onto your back, where you can rest with your knees bent and your feet flat on the bed.

13. Resting in between, have your pelvis spiral you up to sitting and then back down several times, each time remembering:
    - "Spiral,"
    - "Neck end of the body relaxed," and
    - "Reversible."

Sitting Comfortably

It's great if you can buy the perfect chair for yourself—one that encourages you to always have a lumbar curve and allows your feet to be firmly grounded. However, throughout the week you probably sit in many types of chairs in a wide variety of circumstances, so keep the following in mind:

- Allow your pelvis to support your spine. See page 14.

- Always sit on your "sit bones" instead of on your coccyx (especially on a hard bench). See page 39.

- Choose whether or not to lean against the back of a chair remembering that your pelvis can support your posture.

- On a soft couch, put some of the throw pillows behind your back so that the depth of the couch doesn't draw your back into a slouch.

- In a theatre, roll your coat or sweater to make a lumbar support or take your handmade cushion (page 77).

- Be aware of the placement of your feet. Even when you're sitting, that influences how hard the muscles in your back have to work to keep you upright. See page 17.

- Adjust your computer screen so that it encourages a lumbar curve instead of drawing your spine into a slouch.

- Position your reading material so that your head doesn't have to bend over (which bows your spine into a slouch). You can place one or more pillows under a book or magazine to angle your reading material more toward vertical and closer to your eyes.

> **Reminder**: If your lumbar curve is in place, not flattened or slouched, your back and your sciatic nerves will be more comfortable while you're sitting, and also when you stand up after having been sitting for a long time.

Standing Up With Comfort

Every time you come up from sitting to standing—whether in your home, your office, the theater, or a restaurant—take a split-second to organize yourself to prevent joint wear and tear as well as nerve discomfort:

- Your lower back doesn't have to tense or exert effort when your pelvis initiates the movement—instead of having your arms trying to pull you up with your legs and back tightening.

- Reversible springiness—the opposite of rigidity—enables you to move with more comfort through your joints and around your sciatic nerves.

- Knee and foot alignment is very important. You need to have your knees and femoral (hip) joints fully supported by your feet.

Knee and Foot Alignment

Before you stand up, take a split-second to make sure that your knees are aligned with your feet. It's pure skeletal engineering. What's below needs to support what's above.

If your knees are habitually out of alignment with your feet you'll have more wear-and-tear through your joints; your muscles will have to work harder; and your sciatic nerves will be more vulnerable to irritation. This applies whether you're in the process of:

- Coming up to standing from sitting
- Going down to sitting from standing
- Simply standing

Checking Your Knee and Foot Alignment

You can do this experiment with each foot and knee while sitting, and then while standing. With both feet on the ground a comfortable distance apart, place a real, or imaginary, yardstick between your big toe and second toe so that the yardstick is vertical.

1   Notice where your knee is in relationship to the yardstick:

   Is your kneecap outside the yardstick—your knee out wider than your foot?

   Is your kneecap inside the yardstick—your knee in more than your foot?

   Is the inside edge of your kneecap lined up with the yardstick?

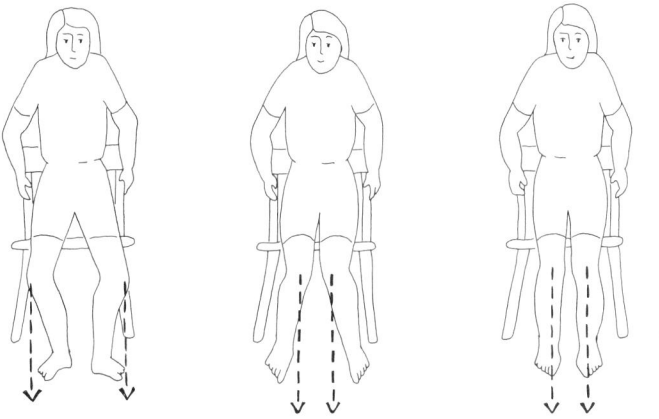

When the inside edge of your kneecap lines up with the yardstick, your knee and foot are in alignment.

Important! Whenever you are standing, about to stand up, or about to sit down—it's very important to have each kneecap centered between the inside edge of your 2nd toe and the outside edge of your 4th toe.

Your Pelvis Is Key In Standing Up Comfortably

When you think skeletally instead of muscularly, your nervous system activates only those muscles needed for the action. As a consequence, you won't be as apt to tighten excessively around your sciatic nerves.

Every bone in your body ultimately connects to your pelvis. If you initiate standing up from your pelvis, you'll be more comfortable. This is especially true if you have a history of sciatica.

An Efficient Way to Stand Up from Sitting

1. Position your feet flat on the ground with each kneecap centered between the inside edge of your 2nd toe and the outside edge of your 4th toe.

2. With your hands on either side of you on the chair (or bed or toilet), have your pelvis and arms lift you closer to the front edge.

3. Let your shoulders and arms relax with your hands resting on either side of you. From this point on, the stronger, lower half of your body will do the work.

4. Decide which leg feels the more reliable at this moment.

    Place that foot so your lower leg can be vertical (perpendicular to the floor).

    Make sure that your kneecap is centered between the inside edge of your 2nd toe and outside edge of your 4th toe.

    Make sure that the foot of your more reliable leg is firmly on the floor, from heel to toes.

5. Move your other foot closer to the chair. As you move this foot back, the front of the foot remains on the ground but your heel will leave the ground so that lower leg will be angled, not vertical.

6. Glue an *imaginary* magnet on your sacrum. Have that "magnet," and your sacrum, lift you up and over your *more reliable* leg.

    The idea of the "magnet" helps you think skeletally instead of muscularly.

    By the time you are fully standing both heels will be on the ground.

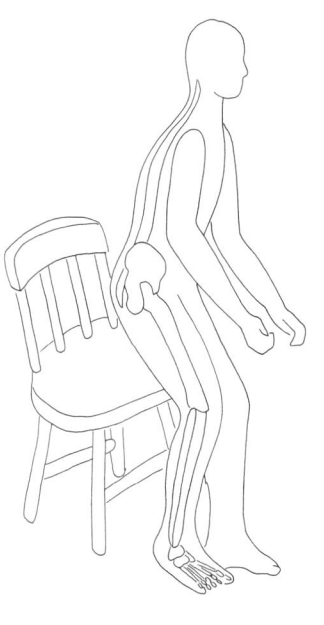

To Sit Down From Standing:

1. Slide the *imaginary* magnet (see pervious page) a bit more toward your coccyx.

2. Have the "magnet" take your coccyx back so that you fold through your hip joints as well as your knees to smoothly sit down.

3. By the time you sit, the heel of your foot that is closest to the chair will leave the ground.

Important! In order to sit down your coccyx has to release backward sooner or later, otherwise all you could do is fall into the chair. To not irritate your sciatic nerves, allow your coccyx to release immediately instead of at the last minute.

Experiment to self-discover if tightening your abdominal muscles helps or interferes:

1. Tighten your abdominal muscle as you stand up from sitting, and then sit down.

2. Now, allow your abdominal muscles to lengthen instead of contract as you stand up from sitting. Then sit back down without tightening your abdominal muscles using the skeletal awareness in the above lesson.

3. Alternate between #1 and #2 so you can discover for yourself if tightening your abdominal muscles actually "puts the brakes on."

Experiment to self-discover if tightening your "gluts" helps or interferes:

1. While standing, tighten your glutei (buttocks) muscles as you try to bend through your knees. Then unbend your knees.

2. Now, relax your glutei muscles as you bend your knees.

3. Briefly alternate between #1 and #2 to confirm for yourself whether or not it really is easier to bend your knees when your glutei muscles are relaxed.

Springy Reversibility

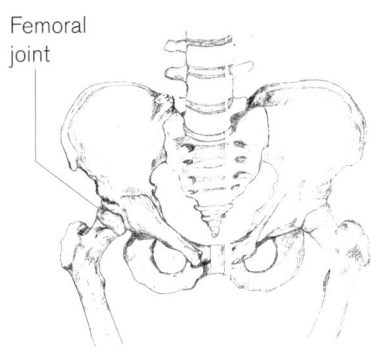
Femoral joint

To smoothly transition from standing to sitting, you need to bend/fold through your femoral (hip) joints, where your legs are ball-and-socketed to your pelvis, not just through your knees. If you don't, you can't sit! To remain comfortable, allow that folding through your hip joints to happen immediately instead of at the last moment Tightening your gluts (even a little bit), which tucks your coccyx (tail bone), prevents easy folding through your hip joints. Instead, allow your coccyx to release backward the moment you begin to sit down.

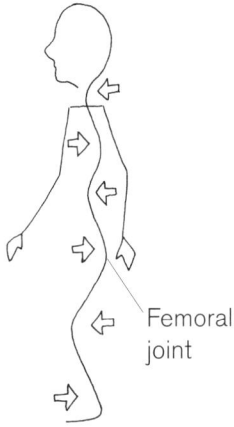
Femoral joint

Important: Tightening the glutei muscles (which tucks the coccyx under) is problematic for everyone, but especially for those with a vulnerability to sciatica. It can happen out of habit with the person only aware of discomfort, not the cause of the discomfort.

Standing at a Counter

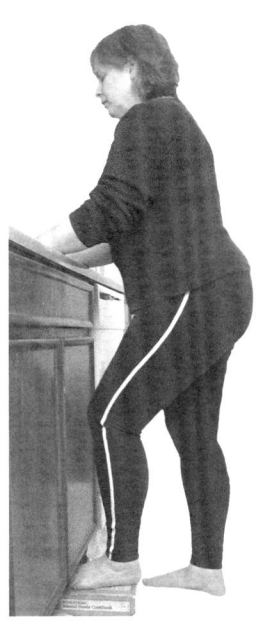

Whether you're standing at your kitchen counter, a counter at work, or a counter in a store—having one foot back a bit will help keep your back more comfortable.
Standing with one foot back –

➢ Encourages a lumbar curve because it discourages dropping the coccyx under

➢ Encourages the sternum (breastbone) to be forward and up, which makes it easier for your arms to work

Standing with your front foot resting on a low footstool or a telephone book encourages your back and your leg to relax as you work.

Bending Over Comfortably, Efficiently

No matter how briefly you're there, every time you bend over you have a choice that can make a difference in the comfort of your sciatic nerves.

> As you bend over, you could drop your coccyx (tail bone) under, which would eliminate your lumbar curve and make your sciatic nerves vulnerable, **or**

> You can do the opposite. That is, release your coccyx backward so that your natural lumbar curve is in place!

As any martial artist knows, your pelvis is your power and balance center—but your pelvis can't do its job if you lock your coccyx under or if you tightly guard your lower back.

Unfortunately, many people consciously make the choice to tuck the coccyx under as they bend over, mistakenly thinking it will help protect the back. Whether done consciously or out of habit, tucking the coccyx as you bend over hurts, not helps, your back and legs.

To keep your sciatic nerves comfortable as you bend over, release your coccyx behind you instead of tucking your coccyx under you. Having one foot back instead of having your feet parallel will encourage you to release, not tuck, your coccyx.

Experiment with Bending Over

1. With your feet parallel and your coccyx tucked a little bit forward and under you, pretend to pick up a tennis ball.

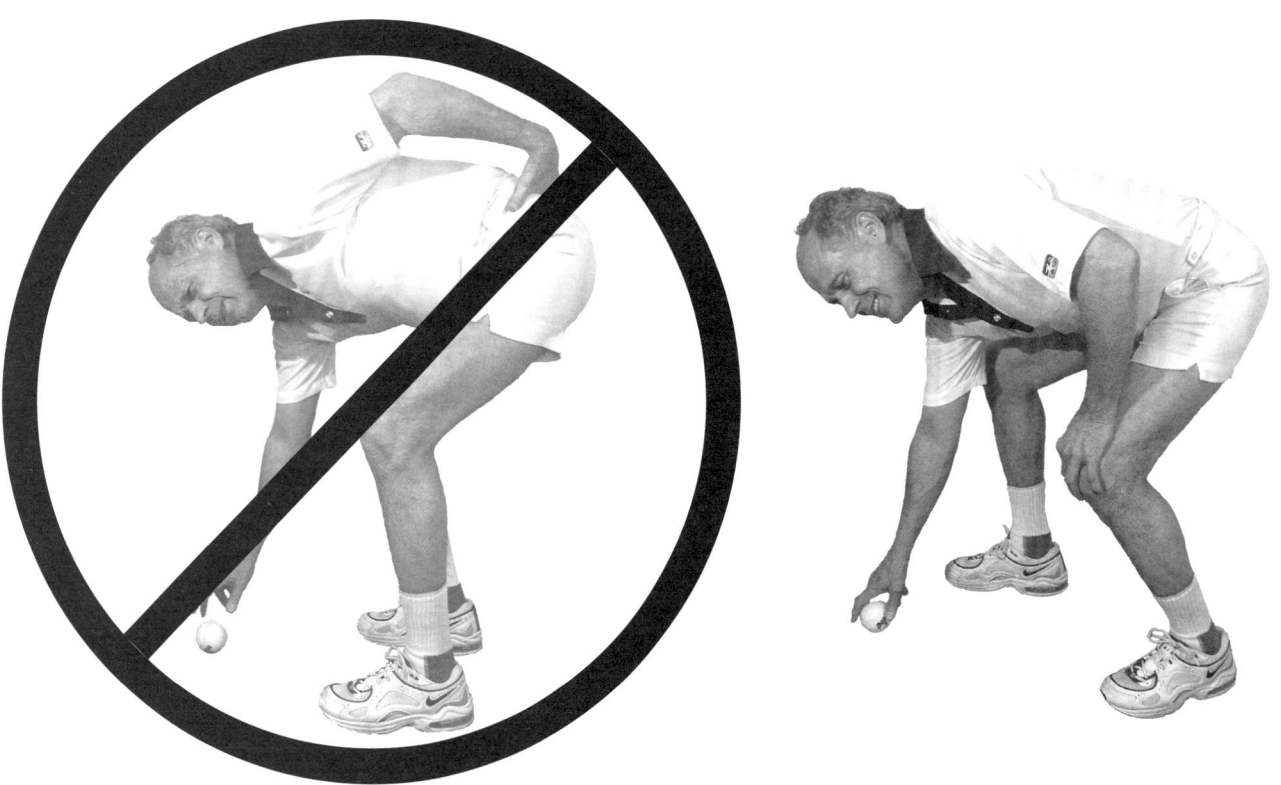

2. Now, with one foot back a little bit and your coccyx released behind you, pretend to pick up a tennis ball again.

3. Alternate between #1 and #2 to confirm:

    Which way was more comfortable for your back?

    Which way was more comfortable for your legs?

    Which way gave your arms more freedom to move?

Tucking your coccyx under is counter-productive to your efficiency and comfort.

Possible consequences include –

- More wear and tear on your hip and knee joints and the nerves that pass through them

- Rounding your spine backward (as your spine is a continuum that includes your sacrum and coccyx).

- Exerting pressure on the front of your spinal vertebrae and the discs that cushion between them

- Compromising the potential flexibility of your spine and the range of motion of your arms

- Wasting muscular effort better spent helping you accomplish your task

Your Personal Progress Notes

8 Walking Can Be Therapeutic

Whether you walk for exercise, to work, up stairs, or only from the kitchen to the living room—walking is a part of your daily life. The choices you make as you walk determine whether you have more, or less, wear and tear through your joints and aggravation through your sciatic nerve network.

Two minor changes in the position of your body as you walk can be major factors as to whether or not your sciatica returns:

➢ How your pelvis is positioned as you walk

➢ How and where your feet contact the ground as you walk

How Your Pelvis Is Positioned

Previous chapters have discussed why trying to protect your back by tucking your coccyx (tail bone) under to flatten your back is not helpful. Unfortunately, many people with chronic sciatica do this while walking.

Flattening your lower back, or tucking your coccyx, while walking actually puts more pressure on your spinal, hip, and knee joints. It also puts more pressure on the sciatic nerves.

Brief EXPERIMENT

1   Briefly, take a few steps while "guarding" or flattening your back.

Note: Flattening your back so that the lumbar curve disappears automatically tucks your coccyx under.

2   Pause and "accordion pleat" (see page 16) to release your coccyx so that it's not tucked under you.

   Notice if you can breathe more easily than when your coccyx is **not** tucked under you.

Notice if you have more comfort through your knees, hip joints, and back when your coccyx is *not* tucked under.

3   Take a few steps without your coccyx tucked under and notice if it is easier and more comfortable to walk this way.

Walking with your coccyx tucked under is like driving your car with the emergency brake on. It causes far more wear and tear. "Unlocking" your coccyx is like taking the emergency brake off.

The importance of how your feet contact the ground

If your heels hit the ground out in front of your torso when you're walking, you can aggravate your joints and sciatic nerves.

To find out if your feet are hitting the ground too far ahead of you, ask yourself these questions:

Does walking aggravate my sciatica and create back or leg pain?

- Do my heels make a noticeable sound when I walk across a wooden floor?
- When I'm on the second floor of the house, can people on the first floor hear me walking?
- Do I have thick calluses on the bottom of my heels?
- Other than calluses on your heels, what are the consequences of habitually having your heels make hard contact with the floor in front of you?
- Walking with your feet hitting the ground out ahead of you may encourage your feet to turn out. If that's the case, your knees and feet are not in alignment as your body weight passes over them
- Walking with your feet hitting the ground out ahead of you can be jarring for your feet, legs, back, and sciatic nerves.

Walking Can Be Theraputic

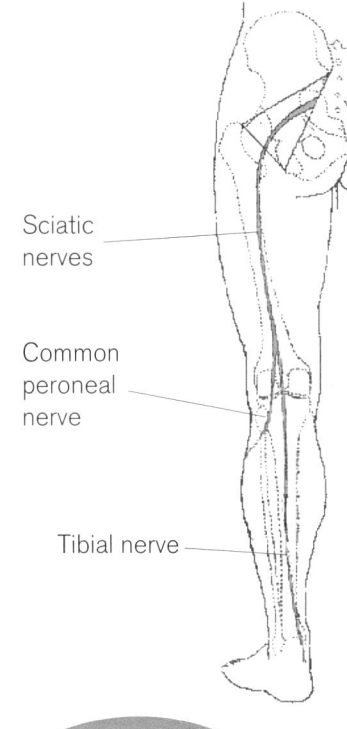

Sciatic nerves

Common peroneal nerve

Tibial nerve

Remember: The tibial nerve (part of your sciatic nerve network) travels from your lumbar vertebrae through the bottom of your femoral (hip) joint, down through the back of each leg, **along the inside edge of each heel**, and down through the arch of each foot. (See page 9.)

The common peroneal nerve (another part of your sciatic nerve network) travels from your two bottom lumbar vertebrae, directly under your femoral joint. Then it branches away from the tibial nerve above each knee, travels along the front of each leg just outside of the tibia (shin bone) and continues **along the outside of each ankle** and over the top of each foot.

Considering the sciatic nerve network's path, can you understand how walking with your heels pounding the ground out in front of you could irritate your sciatic nerves?

At this point you might be thinking, "But I have to get places on time! I don't want to take baby steps!" What's the solution?

You don't have to take tiny steps or walk more slowly—just *allow your stride to be behind you instead of in front of you.* ("Stride" simply is the distance between the front foot and back foot as you're walking.)

Why Walk with Your Stride Behind You?

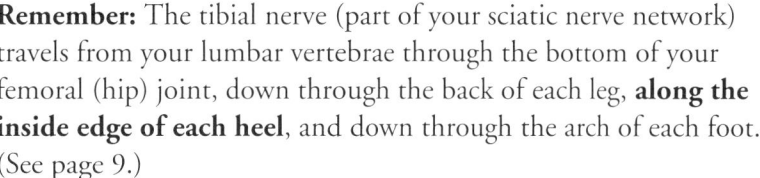

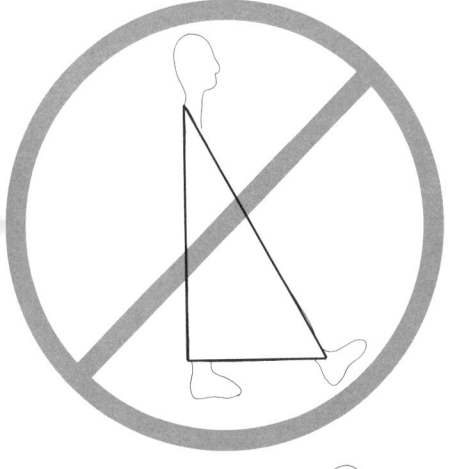

It's purely a learned attitude to think we are more efficient when we stride out ahead. In Western Rehab the focus usually is on getting one foot out ahead and then the other. However, therapists who have had *Feldenkrais* training understand that each foot and leg helps the most when taking its turn **behind,** instead of in front. In societies where people carry water jugs or bundles of wood on top of their heads, they put their stride behind them as they walk.

➢ When each foot takes its turn behind you, it can propel your body forward. (When you stride out ahead of yourself, you can only pull your body forward, not propel your body.)

➢ Having your stride behind you causes less wear and tear on your joints and the nerves threading through them.

> Walking with your stride behind you takes less muscular effort.

> This is the most efficient and most powerful way to walk—on a flat surface, on a hill, or on stairs.

Walking Up Stairs

Equipment needed: One stair or sturdy stepstool or thick book, and a handrail or countertop that you can hold onto for safety and balance

Note: Do not pull with your arms during this experiment; instead, let your legs do the work. Do not tuck your coccyx.

1. Put one foot on the "stair" and have that leg *pull* you up on the stair. Do this several times with the same leg, pausing in between with both feet on the floor.

    Does this feel familiar?

    Notice how much muscular work is necessary for your front leg to *pull* you up the stair.

    Notice if this causes discomfort through your leg or back.

2. Notice that each time your front leg pulls you onto the stair, the heel of your back foot peels off the ground. (It has to or you couldn't continue up the stairs.)

3. Pause and consider the possibility that, instead of the front leg pulling you up the stair, your back foot could **propel** you up the stair since the heel that is behind does have to peel off the ground sooner or later.

4. Consciously allow your back foot to **propel** you forward and up as the heel that is behind you peels off of the ground—instead of the front leg pulling you.

    Don't wait until your front foot is already on the stair. The peeling off the ground by your back heel begins **as** you start to lift your front leg to climb the stair.

    It's the process of the heel leaving the ground that propels your body forward and upward.

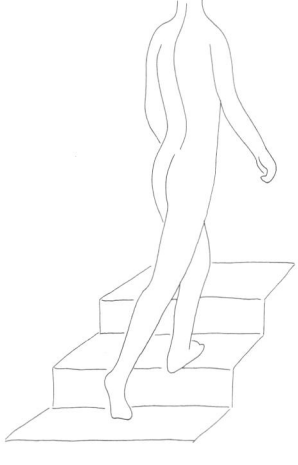

5   Alternate between having your front leg **pull** you up the stair and having your back leg **propel** your body forward and up the stair.

    Notice which way is more efficient for climbing stairs. Notice which way is more comfortable for your body.

Walking With Your Stride Behind You

This experiment will help you discover that the principles you just applied to walking up stairs also apply to walking on a flat surface.

1   First walk a few steps with your stride out in front of you, pulling you forward.

    How much effort does this take?

    How hard do your heels hit the ground?

    Does your center of gravity lag behind your stride?

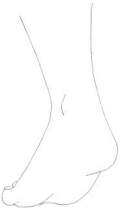

2   Notice that as you walk the heel of whichever foot is in back peels off the ground. (It has to or you couldn't make forward progress unless you shuffle or slide your feet along the ground.)

3   Now, let the heel of your leg that is behind you **propel** you forward as it peels off the ground. This is more efficient than having your front leg and foot *pull* you forward.

    Notice if this actually takes less effort than when your front leg pulled you forward.

    Notice if your heels are not hitting the ground as hard as before.

    Note: Simply use the heel's natural tendency to peel off the ground to help propel your body forward. You don't need to work hard.
    ---

4   When you can differentiate between having your front foot pull you forward and your back foot propel you forward, take a few steps one way and then a few steps the other way.

Observe which way feels more powerful.

Observe which way is more comfortable for your back and legs.

5 Gradually, have whichever foot is in front land right under your body before taking its turn behind you where it propels you forward.

This is what efficient joggers do.

Gradually your stride will be more generous—it will just be behind you instead of in front of you.

Important! When your back leg does the work (instead of your front leg) your walking will be more comfortable, more efficient, more powerful, and more healthful for your nerves and joints.

More About Walking

So far you've seen how the position of your pelvis and where your feet land relative to your body as you're walking can have either a positive or a negative impact on the health of your sciatic nerve network and your hip and knee joints.

Now let's see how the following additional factors can make your walking even more comfortable and healthful:

➢ The mobility of your pelvis—so that your pelvis can help walk your legs

➢ The pliability of your rib basket—so that your spine and pelvis are free to move

Mobility Of Your Pelvis And Spine

If you don't allow your pelvis to rotate while walking, the acetabulum (socket where your leg connects to your pelvis) doesn't move. Instead, only the ball of the femur (thigh bone) moves, forcing your leg to do **all** the work.

Your sciatic nerves thread through the bottom of your femoral (hip) joints; therefore, it's in your best interest to let both the socket and the ball move with every step you take.

Walking Can Be Theraputic

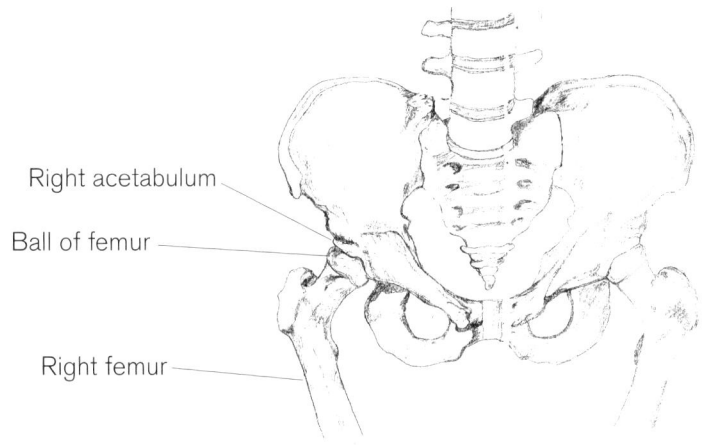

Right acetabulum
Ball of femur
Right femur

Allow your pelvic bowl to subtly rotate to walk your legs. This rotation helps lengthen your stride behind you! As one side of the bowl moves a bit forward, the other side moves backward.

> As your pelvis rotates a bit to the left
>
>> Your right femoral joint moves a little bit forward bringing your right leg with it, and
>>
>> Your left hip moves a bit backward to help your left foot efficiently propel you forward as your left heel peels off the ground.
>
> To take the next step, your pelvis rotates a little bit to the right which:
>
>> Helps your left femoral joint move a bit forward bringing your left leg forward, and
>>
>> Your right hip moves a bit backward to help your right heel take its turn to peel off the ground to propel you forward.

You and your sciatic nerves will be more comfortable if every time you walk — even if it's just across the room — you allow your pelvis to subtly rotate to move your hip joints alternately backward to help each foot power you forward ***while behind you***.

Walking without allowing your pelvis to rotate is like driving your car without the emergency brake released.

Pliability Of Your Rib Basket And Spine

To enable your pelvis to freely help you walk, it's important to have a pliable "rib basket," not a rigid "rib cage." Since half of the mobile vertebrae of your spine have ribs attached, immobilizing your thoracic (rib) vertebrae inhibits comfortable movement through your lower back and pelvis.

Review pages 37–42 to help your rib "cage" become a flexible rib "basket" and the exercise "Regaining A Flexible Spine" beginning on page 49.

A pliable rib basket also helps your arms swing in opposition to your legs for efficient, balanced walking. To facilitate this pliability, wiggle out any tension you hold in your body and let your pelvis power your legs as you **walk with your stride behind you!**

9 Travel Comfortably

This chapter addresses your comfort while traveling by car, plane, bus, or train. The information will help you:

➢ Sit comfortably in a car or public conveyance.

➢ Brake and accelerate comfortably.

➢ Make good use of your time while waiting for a stop light or train.

➢ Twist safely so that you can see to back out of the driveway or talk to the person next to you on a plane, train, or bus.

Sitting Comfortably In Your Car

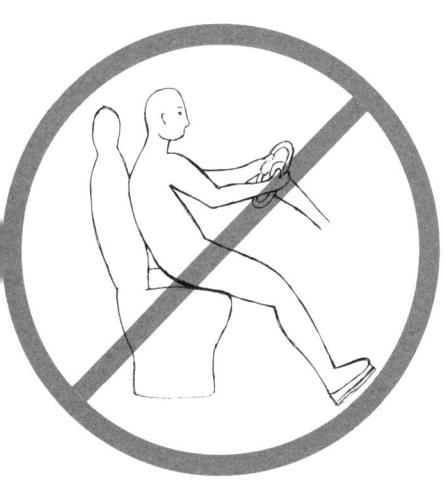

Since it's easy to slide into a slouch while driving — even if your car has a built-in lumbar support — make sure that you scoot your hips back so that your whole sacrum makes contact with the seat back. Whether you're driving a car or only riding in it, you need a supported, relaxed lumbar curve. You also need to ensure that there's no excessive pressure on the back of your thighs or the back of your knees.

Notice how your car's seat fits your body

Sit with your sacrum, your entire back, making contact with the seat back.

Does the back of your car seat support your lumbar curve?

> If it doesn't, you could roll up a towel or some foam rubber and put it in a pillowcase. Place the roll behind you just above your sacrum, in the small of your back, to help you maintain your lumbar curve.

Does your body have to round forward in order for your hands to grasp the steering wheel?

> If so, move the seat forward until you can sit without slouching and have your hands on the steering wheel with your elbows

bent to some degree. (If your car has airbags, there should be about ten inches between your chest and the steering wheel.)

Do you feel pressure under your thighs on your sciatic nerves?

If so, place a soft, flat cushion under your "sit bones" and thighs. (If you're not the driver, you could place a bed pillow under your thighs, which would also help your hips scoot back so that your back is better supported.)

Do you feel pressure under the back of your knees where they contact the front edge of the seat?

If your car seat has electronic controls, use the controls to tilt the front of the seat downward a bit.

Drape an egg-crate foam rubber pad on the car seat under your thighs and a few inches over the front edge of the seat.

Cushion to reduce sciatic nerve pain

Even if your car has plush upholstered seats, the edge of the seat may be exerting pressure against your leg. You can buy, or make, a cushion to take the pressure off the back of your thighs, under the back of your knees, and under your pelvis. This cushion is also helpful when you commute on a bus or train.

Pre-made foam-rubber seat pads with washable covers are available through catalogs and in stores. These are portable and so are also useful for sporting events when you have to sit on a hard bench. However, sometimes pre-made cushions are not long enough or wide enough to take the pressure off the back of the knees while in a car as driver or passenger. The following describes how you can tailor make your own seat cushion.

Make Your Own Seat Cushion

Equipment needed:

Twin-bed size foam-rubber "egg-crate" pad, available at most bedding stores and many discount stores for under $20.

Marking pen or pins, scissors

Optional–pillowcase big enough to cover the finished cushion

1. If using a twin-bed size "egg-crate" foam-rubber pad: place it on your bed lengthwise, matching its lengthwise edge with the edge of your bed.

2. Sit on the above pad with your legs the distance apart they would be if you were actually driving.

3. Mark with a pen or pin on the pad one inch beyond the right side of your right knee and one inch beyond the left side of your left knee.

4. Cut a strip **across** the length of the pad as wide as your markers (probably 1/3 or more of the length of the original "egg-crate" pad).

5. What you just created is a new rectangle. The width of the original rectangle pad is now the length of your new rectangular pad.

6. With the bumpy "egg-crate" side up, wrap this pad a few inches over the front edge of the seat of your car to cushion the underside of your knees. Continue draping the pad over the part you sit on to cushion the underside of your upper legs and pelvis, and part way up to cushion between your lower back and the vertical back of your car seat.

Caution: It may be tricky at first getting into and out of your car with this pad in place, however for those of you vulnerable to sciatic pain this pad is priceless. For long trips you may want to cut two identical strips, placing one on top of the other.

Another option

1. Measure the depth of your car seat. Double the resulting number and add 6 inches.

2. Cut a foam-rubber pad into a strip as long as the number derived in Step 1, and wide enough to cushion the back of both knees while driving.

3. Fold the piece in half and put it into a pillowcase.

4. Place your homemade cushion on the driver's seat so that it extends a little bit over the front edge (to protect the back of your knees), yet touches where the horizontal part of the seat meets the vertical back of the car seat.

Braking and Accelerating

If you experience sciatic pain in the leg you use to accelerate and brake, there are a number of conscious choices that you can make to minimize your vulnerability. It's helpful to recognize what you're *actually* doing; then you can decide whether you're going to *choose* another option.

➤ Become aware of the alignment of the foot and knee you use to accelerate and brake.

➤ Become aware of any habitual curling of your toes as you accelerate or brake.

➤ Become aware of how you position your other leg.

➤ Become aware if you're tightening unnecessarily through your back or hips.

➤ Become aware if you're gripping the steering wheel tighter than necessary with your hands, or unnecessarily tightening your jaw, as both can have repercussions down into your lower back.

Alignment of your foot and knee. If, while driving, your lumbar curve has been supported and you have a cushion between your leg and the seat of the car, but your back or leg still hurts, your knee may be out of alignment with your foot:

➤ Line up the center of your kneecap with your middle three toes.

➤ As you move your foot between the accelerator and brake pedal, rotate your leg from the hip so that your knee can stay aligned with your toes.

➤ Use your footprint to accelerate, i.e. not the arch of your foot.

How your hip joints can help. Tightening excessively through your hip joints can exert unnecessary pressure on the back of your thighs and your sensitive sciatic nerves. Instead, allow your hips, lower back, rib basket, even your shoulders, to relax as much as possible so that your ball-and-socket hip joints don't restrict the movement of your leg(s) as you accelerate or brake.

Relax your toes. Do you habitually grip with your toes (curl your toes under) as you accelerate or brake? This can torque your knee out of alignment with your foot, and cause leg or back pain.

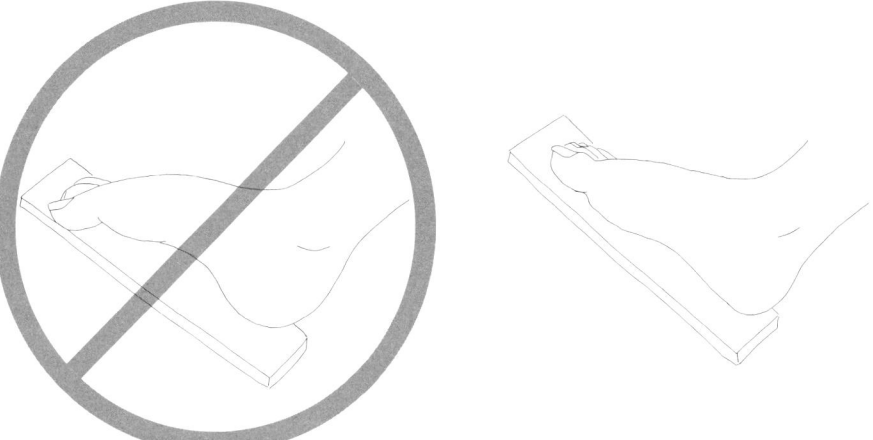

Position of your other leg. Unnecessary tension in either leg causes tension through your hip joints and lower back, Have your other foot make relaxed but firm contact with the floor or on the wheel well.

Waiting for stop lights or trains

Instead of being irritated by any imposed stop, you could view it as an opportunity for "constructive fidgeting" (see Chapter Five) and relaxation. You could –

- ➢ Put your car in park and take your foot off the brake pedal while you wait for a train to pass.

- ➢ Exhale deeply and then breathe into your entire back.

Note: Your lungs are like balloons that expand not just forward, but also out to the sides *and backward*. (See page 26.)

- ➢ Intentionally go into a bit of a slouch and then regain your posture by repositioning your pelvis. (See page 36.)

- ➢ Wiggle side to side through your ribs to snake your spine. (See page 41.)

Sitting and Standing on a Bus, Boat, Plane, or Train

The next time you're on a bumpy bus or a swaying train, notice if you tighten your back or your legs. If you do, your joints and nerves are more vulnerable, not less vulnerable, to jarring.

In some countries where riding horseback is a way of life from childhood on, a person goes riding to relax his or her back at the first sign of back discomfort.

If you relax and let your rib basket and spine "snake" in response to the movement, the swaying and jostling of a bus or train can actually be therapeutic. (See the Side-to-Side Rib Wiggle on page 41).

You have "springs" and "struts" just as your car has springs and struts.

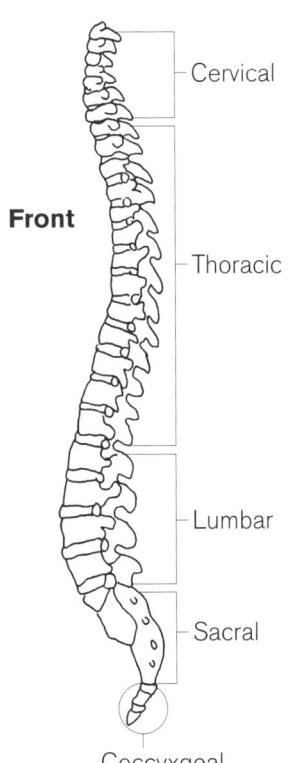

Your "springs" (the moveable vertebrae in your lumbar, thoracic, and cervical curves) cushion up and down motion.

Your "struts" (the ability of your rib basket to asymmetrically "snake" your spine) cushion side-to-side motion.

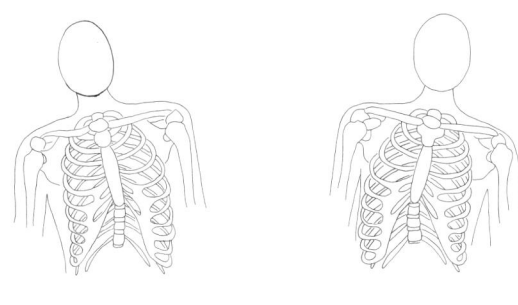

If you freeze your rib "basket" into a rib "cage" and stiffen your spine, you eliminate the internal shock absorbers meant to cushion you.

Turning to See or Talk

Have you been told not to twist because you have a vulnerable lower back? Then how do you look over your shoulder when you're driving?

This book does not suggest that you vigorously twist when in the throes of a sciatica attack. Instead, the following exercise reminds your body that when you even out the distribution of labor, with your lumbar vertebrae passively rotated by the rest of your spine, your lower back is safer.

1. Sit on the edge of your bed, or on a bench or chair that doesn't have armrests.

2. Look over your left shoulder and notice how far you can actually see.

    Notice your comfort level as you look over your left shoulder.

3. This time, let your head and neck be passive and just rotate your rib basket to the left a few times.

    Use your sternum (breastbone in the center front of your rib basket) as a landmark.

    What happened through your neck and head each time you rotate your sternum? Did they also rotate, but passively?

    When your sternum rotates, the section of spine directly below your neck rotates which then rotates your neck.

    Notice that your spine below your rib basket wants to also follow the rotation. Since your spine is a continuum, your rib basket cannot rotate very much unless you allow your lumbar vertebrae and pelvis to follow the rotation.

4. This time, rotate your pelvis a little bit to the left a few times by taking your left hip backward.

    Notice what happens through your whole spine as your pelvis rotates, **if** you don't tighten and try to prevent it.

    Notice if your head rotates each time you rotate your pelvis.

Now you are moving from below your lumbar spine to see over your left shoulder and your lumbar spine can safely, passively go for the ride.

5   As you rotate your pelvis to the left, gently also rotate your sternum to the left.

Notice how far you can see to the left now even though your neck and your lower back just followed passively.

Notice your comfort level as you look over your left shoulder now.

6   When you are ready, complete steps #1 through #5 to your right

10 Resume Activities Confidently

You don't have to live in fear of your pain returning any more than you have to "live with" sciatica pain. The key to resuming activities with confidence and comfort is awareness of how you position your skeleton.

To stop hurting ourselves, we must learn to be aware of what we're doing—not to be oblivious.

This chapter covers only a few select activities, but you can apply the principles to every action in your life.

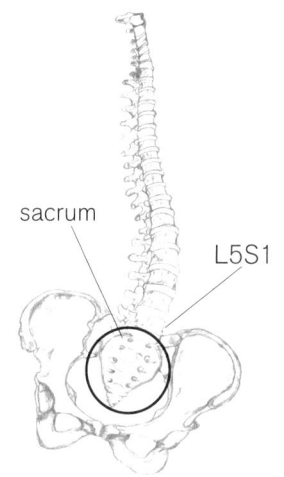

Lifting A Heavy Load

It's common knowledge that bending through your knees as you lift a child, or a heavy load, allows your legs instead of your back to do the work. This is good engineering.
However, if you tuck your coccyx (tailbone) under as you lift:

- ⊘ The resulting subtle slouch of your spine puts pressure on the front of your vertebrae—especially at L5S1 where your bottom lumbar and top sacral vertebrae meet. This is not a good idea, especially when lifting a heavy load. Your sciatic nerve network emerges from the two bottom lumbar vertebrae and the top three sacral vertebrae!

- ⊘ All your weight goes into your knees. The resulting strain can be problematic for your knee joints.

- ⊘ Your balance is more precarious—right when you need it to be the most reliable.

- ⊘ You won't be as strong! (Strength isn't just about muscles; it's also about leverage.)

Healthful way to lift a heavy load

As you do the following exercise, keep these points in mind:

➤ Lengthen your spine (not compact it), during the whole process of bending and lifting.

➤ Keep the load close to your body throughout the lift. The object you lift should follow the line of your spine.

Important! If you tuck your coccyx under while lifting or holding anything, not only will you irritate your sciatic nerves, you won't be as strong. Awareness of your skeletal positioning is extremely useful.

---

1. Instead of flattening your back or tucking your coccyx forward and under, let your coccyx go backward as you bend your knees. This allows you to fold through your femoral (hip) joints more freely and your sternum (breastbone) can remain facing forward, not downward.

2. As you lift, your pelvis moves forward and upward—without your coccyx tucking.

    Your legs are doing the lifting. Your pelvis is the fulcrum, which moves your upper body upright.

3. Do not tuck your coccyx under even when you complete the movement and are standing.

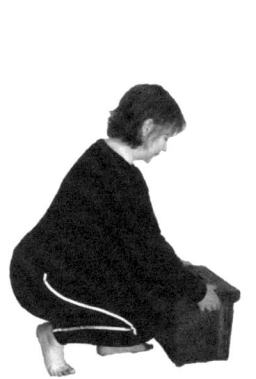
Step 1

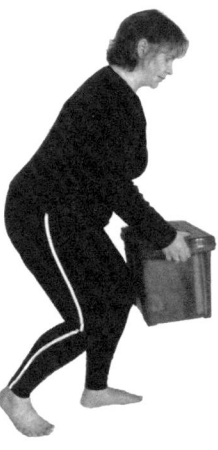
Step 2

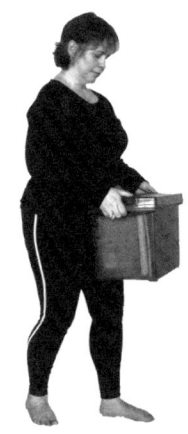
Step 3

Kneeling and Reaching (Gardening)

With your history of sciatica, you may have been avoiding gardening. It's likely that gardening irritated your sciatic nerves *if you guarded or rounded your back*. However, you have another option—allow yourself to have a lumbar curve. Sound familiar?

This next experiment will help you discover that having a lumbar curve not only makes your back more comfortable, it also frees your arm to reach more efficiently.

> You have the option of doing this next experiment (and your actual gardening) while sitting on a stool.

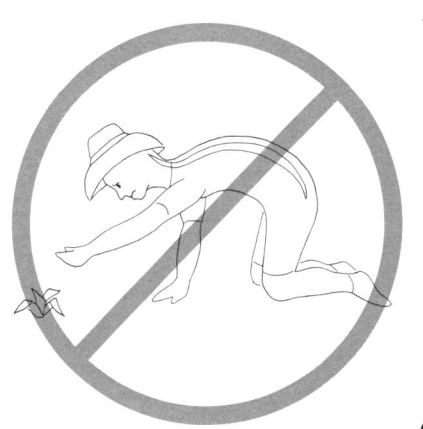

1. *As if you were gardening*, round your back by tucking your coccyx under as you reach out with your hand.

    Reach several different places—out in front of you, to the side, and on a diagonal. Is this comfortable for your body?

    Could you reach very far if you rounded (slouched) your back as you gardened?

2. Now allow yourself to have a lumbar curve as you reach out with your hand. (The key is to **not** tuck your coccyx under.)

    Reach several different places—out in front of you, to the side, and on a diagonal.

    Can you reach farther when you allow yourself to have a lumbar curve?

    Is your back more comfortable?

Riding a Bicycle

Riding a bicycle, whether stationary or regular, has great exercise and therapeutic value. That value can be even greater when you address two factors:

➢ The mobility of your pelvis and spine

➢ The position of your pelvis and spine

At this point you may be thinking, "I thought bicycling was just about legs." Consider the following:

➢ On each side of your body, the sciatic nerve network passes through the bottom of your ball-and-socketed femoral (hip) joint.

➢ If the socket in your pelvis stays stock still, the movement of your leg may irritate your sciatic nerves.

Knowing this, do you really want to keep your pelvis stationary and just pump your legs?

Champion bicyclist Lance Armstrong, multi-time winner of the 3,350 kilometer Tour de France, lets his pelvis move so fast that French sportscasters nicknamed the movement after the rapid wing action of a butterfly.

You don't have to move your pelvis that fast, but do let it move.

As your right leg and foot move forward and down, let your right femoral joint move forward and down. As your left leg and foot move forward and down, let your left femoral joint move forward and down.

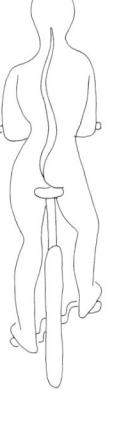
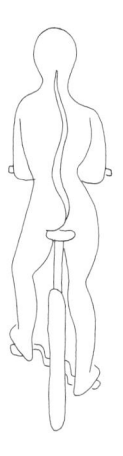

As one side of your pelvis goes forward and downward, the other side passively goes backward and upward. You can't move one side of your pelvis without moving the other.

➢ Your pelvis can drive your legs like pistons.

➢ When the "socket" and the "ball" move together, you're less likely to irritate your hip joints and sciatic nerves.

➢ Allow your rib "cage" to be a pliable rib "basket" so that it doesn't trap your spine and, therefore, trap your pelvis.

First Bicycle Experiment

Next time you're on your bicycle, try this experiment.

1. Briefly, without letting your pelvis, ribs, or spine move, make your legs do all the work.

2. Then, as another brief experiment begin to allow your pelvis to move, but still keep a stiff rib "cage."

3. Stop and wiggle out your ribs to encourage a rib "basket." (See page 41.)

4. As you resume bicycling, let your ribs be free to move from side to side, so that:
   - Your spine can snake side-to-side.
   - Your pelvis is free to power your legs.

Second Bicycle Experiment

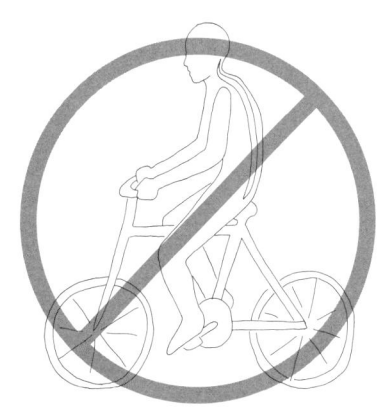

If you enjoy the idea of bicycling, but don't feel good after actually going for a ride, you may be rounding your back, which takes the lumbar curve away and interferes with the movement of your spine and pelvis.

1. As a brief experiment, round or slouch your back while you *try* to allow your spine to snake so that your pelvis can power your legs.

   How easily can you move your pelvis and ribs when you're in a slouch?

2. Instead of rounding your back, rearrange your pelvis to give yourself a lumbar curve. (See page 14.)

   Notice if this second way frees up your ribs and spine so that your pelvis can be more mobile to power your legs.

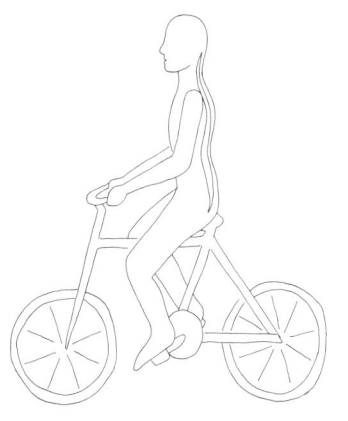

3. Now think of your spine as lengthening up from your pelvis to the top of your neck—in a relaxed way, of course, so your rib basket can still be mobile.

Note: If you have a bike with low handlebars: fold forward through your femoral (hip) joints to reach the handles (instead of slouching) to let your spine lengthen up through your neck.

Relaxing At The End Of The Day

If your pain begins to return after an hour or so of reading or watching TV, you may think it's something you did earlier in the day that caused the pain. ***However, the position of your skeleton-- while you relax, read, or watch TV-- may be the culprit!***

- Reading with your newspaper or book on your lap may tilt your head and neck forward rounding your spine into an unintended slouch. (Look at the bottom of this page for more healthful option.)

- Having your legs suspended between the chair and a footstool may hyperextend your knees. This hyperextension could irritate the tibial nerve (part of the sciatic nerve network) as it passes through the center back of each knee.

- Sitting with your spine in a slouch, which rounds your natural lumbar curve backward, makes you vulnerable. This position and gravity put extra pressure on the front of your lumbar vertebrae, the discs between those vertebrae, and your sciatic nerves.

Remember: Your sciatic nerve network originates from the 4th and 5th lumbar vertebrae and the 1st, 2nd, and 3rd sacral vertebrae—the very region that's most vulnerable when slouching.

Remember: The human skeleton is engineered for sitting on the ischial tuberosities ("sit bones"), not on the coccyx or sacrum. (See page 36.).

It's really all quite logical. You will be more comfortable *and* more effective if you apply "skeletal engineering" to all of your activities.

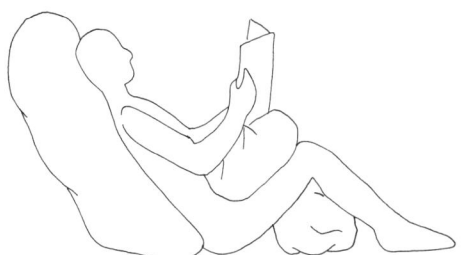

Roll to Relax

This last exercise –

➢ Encourages you to roll from your side to your back and then return to your side again in the most efficient and comfortable way

➢ Improves the circulation through your entire back, hip joints, and legs

➢ Can be very relaxing and calming for your sciatic nerves

Equipment needed: A pillow for your head and a comfortable place to lie down, wide enough for you to spread your arms at approximately shoulder height (your bed or a mat on the floor)

1   Lie on whichever side is the most comfortable for you today. Place a pillow under your head.

2   Bend your knees so that your top leg can rest on your bottom leg. Bend your elbows so that your top arm can rest on your bottom arm.

3   Allow your whole body, including your jaw, to give in to gravity.

4   Several times, roll your body a little bit backward and then forward as if you were going to roll onto your back, but then changed your mind.

> Where did you start the rolling? Was it in your arms and upper body?

5   Let your upper body (including your neck) relax, so that **your pelvis can passively roll your upper body**.

Important! Your whole body will be more comfortable if you initiate movement from your pelvis—*even if* (especially if) you are in the midst of sciatica.

---

6   Think of moving from your sacrum (the section of your spine in the center back of your pelvis) as you allow your pelvis to roll you a little bit backward and then forward.

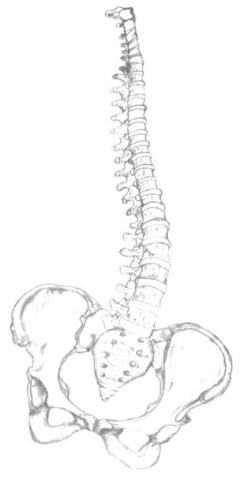

7 As a brief experiment, make your muscles work to roll your pelvis.

> Does tightening muscles in your lower back or buttocks help you or does it just cause discomfort through your back and legs?

Note: For the rest of this exercise, think skeletally not muscularly. When thinking muscularly, most people activate muscles unnecessary to the action. However, when you think skeletally, your central nervous system activates *precisely* the muscles necessary for the movement. It's more therapeutic and more efficient!

8 This time think **skeletally** as your pelvis slowly rolls your body backward and forward.

> Because your sacrum and coccyx are actually part of your spine, your pelvis is a powerful handle by which to roll your spine and all that is attached.

9 Briefly, as an experiment, keep your top knee snugly against the bottom knee so that the leg can't move.

> Did that trap your pelvis and keep it from being able to roll?

> Because your legs are connected to your pelvis, you need to allow top leg to passively follow the movement of your pelvis in order to not interfere.

10 Allow your top knee to slide on your bottom leg as it is gently tugged by the rolling of your pelvis.

11 Rest for a moment with the awareness that every bone in your body ultimately connects to your pelvis.

12 Resume rolling your body from your pelvis—a bit backward and then forward. Do this several times while noting the following connections:

> ➢ Your neck and head can be rolled from your pelvis because your cervical (neck) vertebrae are part of your spine which is being rolled by your pelvis.

Resume Activities Confidently

> Your shoulder can be rolled by your pelvis because your spine is the center back of your rib basket, and your clavicle ("collar bone") connects your shoulder to your sternum (breastbone), which is the center front of your rib basket.

13. Without lifting your head or pushing with your arms, gradually have your pelvis roll you all the way over onto your back.

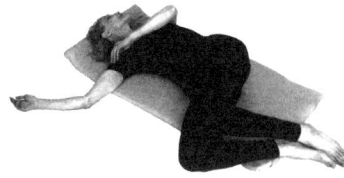

14. Let your arms trail like spaghetti as they follow your sternum which is being rolled by your pelvis.

15. While resting on your back with your knees bent and feet resting on the floor, notice how comfortable you are.

    Was this way of moving from your side onto your back easier as well as more comfortable than your usual way?

16. As you have your pelvis roll you on to your other side, let your arms lazily rest on your chest.

    Don't lift your head or push with your elbows. Instead, simply let your pelvis roll your whole body until you are on your side with your knees bent and resting on the floor.

17. Let your whole body, including your lower jaw, give in to gravity on this side.

18. When you're ready, let your pelvis roll you onto your back, and then over onto your other side so that you can lazily roll from side-to-side.

This author truly hopes *Stop Sciatica Now* empowers you to make healthful movement choices to live pain free.

Pamela

For more information about the *Feldenkrais Method®* of *Somatic Movement Education*, or to locate a *Guild Certified Feldenkrais Practitioner*^{CM} in your area, contact the *Feldenkrais Guild® of North America*:

Visit www.feldenkraisguild.com

E-mail membership@feldenkraisguild.com

Call 1-800-775-2118

For more books by Pamela Kihm visit…
http://www.painfreechoices.com

About the Author

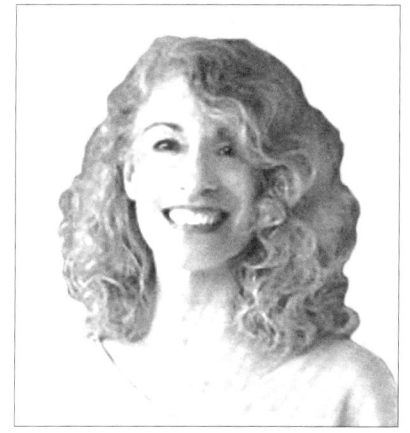

Through the writing of books such as Stop Sciatica Now, and her private practice as a *Guild Certified Feldenkrais Practitioner*[CM], Pamela Kihm's goal is to help people understand healthful movement choices.

With a background as a recreational therapist and exercise teacher, and a degree in Behavioral Science, Pamela had been motivating clients to choose more comfortable options even before completing the 800 hour *Feldenkrais Method® of Somatic Education Professional Training* in 1991. Pamela was one of the first exercise teachers to create "low-impact aerobics" with dances she choreographed so that her students could reach aerobic levels without creating joint damage.

As a *Feldenkrais Practitioner* and exercise trainer for people with challenges, Pamela not only ameliorates symptoms of pain, she helps clients learn how they can move in ways that are more efficient and cause less wear and tear on their bodies. Pamela's clients discover how small modifications to regimens prescribed by the medical community can make exercises even more effective and pain-free.

You can address e-mail to Pamela at pamela@painfreechoices.com

Glossary

Anatomical illustrations pages 7–11, 14–15, 36, 50, 62, 73, 80, 83

"accordion pleat"	bend slightly at the hip, knee, and ankle joints (page 16)
acetabulum	part of *pelvis*; the socket of each ball-and-socket hip joint
"acture"	Moshe Feldenkrais' term for posture (page 16)
cervical curve	healthful spinal curve through neck
cervical vertebrae	bones in the neck; top seven vertebrae of spine
coccyx	tailbone, located at the bottom of your *sacrum*
common peroneal nerve	part of the *sciatic nerve network*
coccygeal vertebrae	bottommost vertebrae of spine, the *coccyx*
Feldenkrais Method®	somatic education method developed by Moshe Feldenkrais
femoral joints	ball-and-socket joint where the *femur* (thigh bone) meets the *acetabulum* (socket) in your pelvis
femur	thigh bone; the "head" of the femur is the "ball" of each hip joint
fulcrum	support on which a layer rests or about which it turns when raising a weight, e.g. *pelvis*
glutei muscles	large muscles in the buttock; includes the gluteus medius, gluteus maximus, and the gluteus minimus
hyper-extended knee	knee so straight that it actually bends a bit backwards
ilium (ilia, *plural*)	hip bone; the uppermost right and left sides of the pelvic bowl
iliac crest	top edge of each *ilium* or *hipbones*
ischial tuberosity	"sit bones;" part of each *ischium* that should bear person's weight when sitting
ischium (ischia, plural)	right and left bottommost part of the pelvis

lengthen	most muscles lengthen by relaxing
lumbar curve	healthful spinal curve through the lower back
lumbar vertebrae	lowest five mobile vertebrae in the spine; above the *sacrum*
pelvis	bony structure shaped somewhat like a bowl which includes the *acetabulum, coccyx, ilium, iliac crests, ischium, sacroiliac joints,* and *sacrum*
piriformis muscle	muscle deep within the buttock, under the gluteus muscles
sacral vertebrae	fused section of the spine in the center back of the pelvis
sacrum	center back of the *pelvis*; the *sacral vertebrae*
sacroiliac joints	where the *ilia* connect to the right and left of sacrum
sciatic nerve network	consists of the tibial and common peroneal nerves and their branches; originates in the lumbar and sacral regions of the spine, threads through the bottom of each hip joint, down each leg, and ends in each foot
shorten	most muscles shorten or contract when tightened
sternum	"breastbone;" center front of the chest, which is connected to the spine by ribs
stride	distance between front foot and back foot while walking
tailbone	bottom of spine; *coccygeal vertebrae* fused to sacrum
thoracic curve	curve in spine located below the *cervical curve* and above the *lumbar curve*, curved in opposite direction of cervical and lumbar curves
thoracic vertebrae	the twelve spinal vertebrae that have ribs attached
tibial nerve	part of the *sciatic nerve network*
vertebra (vertebrae)	bone(s) of the spine
vertebral discs	cushions between the vertebrae of your spine

Index of Lessons

Chapter 1
Touch Your Toes with More Comfort and Ease, 5

Chapter 2
Posture From the Bottom Up, 14
Foot Placement Is Important, 17
Therapy While You Sleep, 20

Chapter 4
Sitting Inch Worm, 23
Standing Inch Worm, 24
Relax around Your Sciatic Nerves, 26
Knee to Chest, 27
Less Is Better Than More—Version I, 30; Version II, 31
Cradle Your Leg, 32

Chapter 5
Intentional Slouching as a Technique, 36
Gentle Side-folding Through Your Ribs, 37
Sitting Gentle Spine Stretch, 38
Standing Gentle Spine Stretch, 39
Side-to-Side Rib Wiggle, 41

Chapter 6
Walk Backward—technique to relax excessive muscular tension, 43
Cat/Camel with Skeletal Awareness, 44
Free Your Upper Back/Help Your Lower Back, 46
Roll to Iron out Your Back, 48
Flexible Rib Basket/Flexible Spine, 49

Chapter 7

Before You Get Out of Bed—reminder of four techniques, 54
Sitting Up From Lying Down, 55
Lying Down From Sitting, 56
Check Your Knee and Foot Alignment, 59
An Efficient Way to Stand Up from Sitting, 60
To Sit Down from Standing, 61
Discover If Tightening Your Abdominal Muscles Helps or Interferes, 61
Discover If Tightening Your "Gluts" Helps or Interferes, 61
Experiment with Bending Over, 64

Chapter 8

Position of Your Pelvis While Walking, 67
Walking Up Stairs, 70
Walking with Your Stride Behind You, 71

Chapter 9

Make Your Own Seat Cushion, 77
Turning to See or Talk, 81

Chapter 10

Lifting a Heavy Load, 84
Kneeling and Reaching (Gardening), 85
Riding a Bicycle, 87
Roll to Relax, 89